Contents

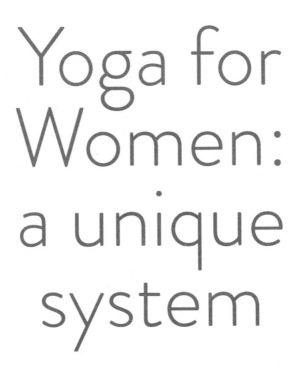

Yoga for Women: a unique system

In today's society, women have lifestyles that make it necessary for them to be ever more active, more yang. We have endless 'to-do' lists at work, as well as at home. We desire to 'succeed': as a perfect woman, a perfect mother, a perfect colleague, and we hope to achieve personal and professional goals. We manage it, but at what price? Stress and exhaustion, both physical and emotional.

The methods described in this book are the result of my personal quest for sacred femininity and inner peace, so that every woman can respect her own rhythm and take care of her body.

A woman's well-being is linked to her menstrual cycle, which undulates like a sine wave. Women are predisposed to the influence of the endocrine system and nature, and have mood swings linked to hormonal changes.

It is therefore fundamental for women to understand every stage of their hormonal cycle, as well as the feminine life cycle, in order to adapt to and accept it with goodwill.

I was born into a family where femininity and sexuality were never discussed. The 'camaraderie' of the Soviet Union doubtless influenced the women in my family and, by extension, me. At the age of 20 I felt the need to live in my woman's body and reconnect with my femininity. I explored 'soft' methods: yoga, meditation, acupressure, qi gong and so on. I learned to listen to myself, to connect to the real me. I discovered my deepest desires and needs and I stopped wanting to simply please others. Little by little, I understood how to value myself, to please myself and to be myself. These days, each time I practise, it instils in me a little more inner calm, emotional stability and feminine joy.

Over more than ten years of teaching yoga, I learned from the experiences of the women I met. My observations grew into Yoga for Women, a complete method that meets the physiological needs of women, which I have taught since 2014. I aimed to create an approach that boosts energy, lifts the spirits, discharges negative emotions and awakens the gentleness and femininity of every woman.

I am delighted to see women of all ages and from all countries blossoming. I hope that women rediscover and re-centre themselves in the 'being' and forget the 'doing'.

What is Yoga for Women?

This fully comprehensive method encompasses the fundamental philosophies of the main schools of yoga, traditional medicines from China and India, alternative medicines and shamanistic practices.

Through the use of Hatha yoga postures, facial yoga, hormone yoga therapy, Luna yoga, Yin yoga and Restorative yoga, the method stimulates different organs, chakras, energy channels and acupressure points in order to achieve an energy balance that is fundamental to Indian holistic disciplines and traditional Chinese medicine.

I also included some Russian shamanistic practices such as visualisation and rotation, for mental and physical well-being.

Finally, I added some introductions to alternative medicines like naturopathy and crystal healing to complete the practice.

It is thanks to these associations that Yoga for Women will connect you to your femininity, to your gentleness, and to your emotional, physiological and physical well-being.

As you practise it, you can live all the stages in the life of a woman: periods, pre-menstrual, pregnancy, post-childbirth, pre-menopause and menopause. You can stabilise your cycle and balance your hormonal and energy systems. You will enjoy a calm mind, awakened sexuality and inner and outer beauty.

Yoga for Women is for women:

- of all ages;
- who have hormonal problems (menstrual cramps, mood swings, skin complaints etc.);
- who are going through the menopause or are post-menopausal;
- who have infertility issues;
- who seek emotional stability;
- who wish to develop their femininity and sexuality;
- who want to increase their general well-being;
- who are unable to let go and are hyperactive.

As you practise Yoga for Women, don't be a perfectionist. Let yourself go; appreciate and savour the precious moments of connecting with yourself.

Four concepts

When you practise Yoga for Women, embrace your weaknesses and remember that you are perfect as you are. Explore yourself without judging and apply these four concepts.

Total self-acceptance: This is not a simple task for the majority of women who have grown up in an environment of criticism, expectation and blame. Even if the intentions were sometimes benevolent, each sentence or observation is not without consequence on our psyche: criticism can sometimes develop throughout a lifetime and manifest itself in mental repetition (conscious or unconscious). Be positive and lead yourself sympathetically towards a place where destructive criticism does not exist.

Understand your needs: Certain needs are universal, like being loved, respected and understood, for example. Others depend upon the individual: to be part of a couple or not, have children or not, to pursue a career etc.

Women often confuse their own needs with those of society, their culture or those close to them. It is therefore often the case that these societal needs have nothing to do with their actual needs.

In order to understand your own needs, be introspective. Take the time to ask yourself what you like and what you really want, and also what you don't want, or no longer need.

Listen to your body: According to Danièle Flaumenbaum[1], most women are 'split in two' by pressure from society. This rift is situated at waist level and marks the frontier between the top and bottom of the energetic body. Energy that is stuck in the top of the body prevents natural flux movement and creates an excess of masculine energy. On a physical and emotional level, this translates as an inability to listen or be in tune with your bodily sensations and may cause sexual insensitivity. In order to avoid this, listen to yourself and take time for yourself.

Respect your limits: This is linked to all three of the preceding concepts. It is important for women to accept that they owe nothing to anyone. Each woman has her own story and her own limits. The quicker the assimilation, the easier it will be to respect physical, emotional, mental and spiritual boundaries.

---

1   Danièle Flaumenbaum, *Woman Desired, Woman Desiring,* Aeon Books 2020.

The tools

Postures in yoga are directly linked to energy centres known as **chakras**. They strengthen or relax the body and stimulate an organ or endocrine gland.

Exercises in facial yoga enable the firming up and relaxing of the muscles in the face, shoulders and neck and, by extension, the whole body.

Mudras – the specific positioning of the hands – and **breathing exercises**, **meditation** and **visualisation** serve to re-centre and channel the mind for healing and concentrating on the essentials.

Sankalpa, the powerful intention

Sankalpa signifies 'a wish connected to a higher truth'. It is an intention that takes root in the real desires of your heart and which calls to a superior strength in order to incite a change in you.

At the start of a session, you can pronounce your *sankalpa* as a wish: a resolution to guide your practice towards making a better version of yourself. This serves the purpose of making a connecting thread for the whole session. In this way, each posture and breath may feed that intention. It is also possible to repeat the *sankalpa* at the end of a session to make the most of the mental and physical healing to reinforce the wish.

You are welcome to create or modify my proposed intentions at the start of each session if they do not fit completely with your deeper personal intentions. To create your own *sankalpa*, it must:

- be positive and not negative ('I am blossoming' and not 'I don't want to be unhappy anymore');

- be in the present or in the past ('I am buying/I bought the house of my dreams' and not 'I will buy the house of my dreams');

- be related to you ('My relationship with my son is a good one' and not 'My son will understand and will change his attitude towards me').

Asanas – liberating postures

Postures, or *asanas* in Sanskrit, signify 'a position which is comfortable' – that is to say being present and connected with your own body.

Accompanied by breathing and supported by the intention, postures allow a reconnection to the present and favour a better understanding of yourself.

Each posture cleanses the body and mind. A sequence of postures, like a dance routine, enables you to freely express yourself in joy or sadness, and to discover a state of bliss and freedom.

More dynamic postures will require greater physical effort. They will awaken the masculine strength necessary to take your life back into your own hands. It is mainly upright and sitting positions that strengthen muscles, sharpen the mind and refill energy reserves.

Gentler postures connect with sacred femininity through their slowness and softness. They often take place on the floor, sitting or lying, and soothe through their link to the earth. They also stimulate the opening of the hips, improve the circulation of energy in the lower body and reactivate female power. They favour letting go, acceptance and calm.

Yoga for Women mainly uses gentle postures to connect you with your female energy. Listen to your body and your heart during this journey into yourself. Let yourself be guided towards healing and well-being by creating your own postures, which will respect your own level of stiffness, your abilities, and your feelings.

Chakras, vortexes of life

Chakras were identified thousands of years ago by practitioners of yoga and other energy-channelling disciplines. The word 'chakra' means 'vortex', meaning a funnel of energy that takes root in the spine or in the head in order to leave the body.

The body that we are used to seeing is not the only part of our psycho-spiritual existence. It would be better to imagine ourselves with layers, like a Russian doll. The smallest doll represents our physical body (the one we see and touch). The largest doll would be our spiritual being (the mind). The central doll would be the subtle body (where the chakras are located), that is itself made up of three layers: energetic, mental and higher mental. It is in the energetic layer of the subtle body that chakras are located, flowing clockwise at their own speed. Although they are invisible, it is easy to feel their energy (often as a warm feeling in the hands).

Chakras are located all along the spine. The lowest is the root chakra, level with the coccyx. The highest is the crown chakra, at the top of the skull.

Yoga for Women follows the model of tantric yoga[2], which focuses mainly on the seven major chakras, which are responsible for our anchoring (our base, our support) in the material world and for our spiritual development. Their main

---

2 As proposed by Arthur Avalon at the end of the twentieth century and based on the Hindu text *Sat Chakra Nirupana*.

function is to replenish energy and to integrate it into the mind–body and to flush out used energy (negative thoughts, undigested emotions, psychological trauma etc.)

Chakras are very important in the practice of Yoga for Women, as the postures during each session act on one or more chakras linked to organs, feelings or emotions. The postures have been chosen to stimulate or activate different chakras in order to regain a balance of energy.

Root chakra

Colour: red
Physical placement: between the anus and genitals
Associated organs: bones, skeleton, legs, feet, coccygeal plexus, perineum, colon, genitals, adrenal gland
Function: connection with the material world, anchoring
Issues: insecurity, survival

The first chakra, or root chakra – *muladhara* in Sanskrit – is situated at the level of the coccyx. It is responsible for the well-being of the lower body and the organs that are situated there. Its location in the pelvis means it is very important for the health and well-being of women.

The root chakra is linked to the two chakras that are located in the feet that help with our connection to the earth. Its energy and properties allow us to connect better with our body, to feel welcome and safe in the world.

If your root chakra is balanced:
You are stable, patient, relaxed, serene. You feel good and have the sensation of being in a good place at the right time. You speak with confidence. You appreciate your body as it is and you take care of it. You are generous and prosperity conscious. You trust others and you trust life. You are healthy and full of energy. You accept life as it comes and you rejoice in it. You make the most of stable situations across all areas: work, relationships, accommodation. Money is not a source of worry.

If your root chakra is unbalanced:
You are often scared. You feel abandoned, disconnected, vulnerable. You feel as if you do not fit in the world or as if you are not worthy. You are 'overcontrolling'. You play the role of victim; you are hostile, mistrustful. You feel as if you are invisible. You do not like your body as it is. You are under the impression that you need to prove yourself worthy of succeeding. Financial security is a significant preoccupation.

To activate your root chakra:
- Have a foot massage
- Have a running race
- Walk barefoot through grass
- Do some gardening
- Wear red clothes
- Sort your finances
- Engage in anchoring techniques
- Use this positive affirmation: 'I have the right to exist because I was born.'

Sacral chakra
Colour: orange
Physical placement: between the pubis and the bellybutton
Associated organs: sex organs, ovaries, uterus, sacral plexus, bladder
Function: connection with others, creativity, growth
Issues: closure, obsession, lack of sexual relations

The second chakra – *svadhisthana* in Sanskrit – or the sacral chakra, is situated in your energy body at the level of your lower abdomen, between the pubis and the bellybutton.

The sacral chakra is essential in the blossoming of a woman because it is responsible for the well-being of the organs of the lower abdomen, including the ovaries and the uterus. It plays an important role in the circulation of female energy. It influences pleasure and creativity.

If your sacral chakra is balanced:
You are happy, satisfied, relaxed, charismatic, creative and emotionally independent. You love to communicate and share. You appreciate and feel as if you are worthy of attention and wealth. For you, sex is a way of sharing joy with your partner. Those close to you feel good in your presence. You make the most of the simple things in life. You are creative in all areas of your life.

If your sacral chakra is unbalanced:
You feel alone, anxious, abandoned, dependent, ashamed and angry with the opposite sex. You feel like a victim. You talk a lot to earn attention. You put up personal barriers. You don't want anyone to touch you. Making love is difficult, or you do it without feeling. Every small obstacle becomes a difficulty that you lack the creativity to overcome.

To activate your sacral chakra:
- Have a bath
- Have a massage
- Eat good, hot food
- Swim
- Wear orange clothes
- Get enough sleep
- Use this positive affirmation: 'My sexuality and my creativity are emerging into this world.'

Solar plexus chakra
Colour: yellow
Physical placement: solar plexus
Associated organs: solar plexus, digestive system and organs, kidneys, pancreas
Function: courage, action, confidence, power
Issues: excessive power or control

The third chakra – *manipura* in Sanskrit – or the solar plexus chakra, is situated at the level of the solar plexus and is responsible for the digestive organs and the pancreas. This chakra is linked to inner strength and confidence. Its energy enables us to pursue our life projects.

It is often underused by women who are overloaded with tasks at home and in the workplace. This underactivity transforms the energy into 'masculine energy'.

If your solar plexus chakra is balanced:
You feel powerful and want to use that power to achieve good things. You are open to different opinions and are ready to make adjustments. You are well organised, active, motivated and honest. You are responsible for your own actions, courageous and you are invested in your life purpose.

Your digestive system works perfectly and you rarely have stomach problems.

If your solar plexus chakra is unbalanced:
If this energy centre is spent, you feel powerless. People and events take control of you. You get anxiety-related stomach aches. You are frightened of power and prefer it if others take decisions for you. Your lack of self-confidence means you often ask others what they think of you.

If this energy centre has too much energy, you have a thirst for power and are egocentric. You like to feel superior to others. You get angry quickly. You are hyperactive, stressed and you try to do too much in too little time.

To activate your solar plexus chakra:
- Make an open fire
- Work on your abs
- Do some abdominal exercise
- Sunbathe
- Laugh
- Make decisions quickly
- Use this positive affirmation: 'I am the source of my own power.'

Heart chakra
Colour: green
Physical placement: centre of the chest
Associated organs: cardiac, respiratory, lymphatic and immune systems, thymus, arms and hands
Function: devotion, love, detached connections
Issues: lack of love

The fourth chakra – *anahata* in Sanskrit – or the heart chakra, is found at heart level, at the centre of the chest, and is responsible for the lungs, the heart and blood circulation. It is therefore the 'energetic heart'.

The heart chakra influences relationships, notably with the self. It allows love, understanding and compassion to circulate freely in yourself and towards others. The energy from this chakra can heal the deepest wounds.

If your heart chakra is balanced:
You are full of love and understanding of others and yourself. You feel light, free and detached. You are comfortable with your relationships. You appreciate others for what they are, without trying to change them.

If your heart chakra is unbalanced:
Dysfunction manifests itself in difficult relationships, notably with family or in a couple. Relationship issues bring up old wounds from the past, blocking the passage of energy. As a result of this you do not wish to engage and you overprotect yourself. You are constantly suspicious of others and do not let anyone get near to you. Conversely, you are starved of love and cannot get enough. You try to compensate for this lack of love with an excessive attachment to those close to you, but they are exhausted by this dependence.

To activate your heart chakra:
- Have your hands massaged
- Keep a gratitude journal
- Tell yourself 'I love you' in front of a mirror
- Make tender gestures to those closest to you
- Do some voluntary work.

Throat chakra
Colour: blue
Physical location: throat
Associated organs: vocal chords, mouth, throat, ears, respiratory system, thyroid and parathyroid glands
Function: communication, self-expression, purification
Issues: sending and receiving information, self-expression

The fifth chakra – *vishuddha* in Sanskrit – or the throat chakra, is situated at the level of the throat and is responsible for the thyroid, parathyroid and the throat. It influences self-expression. The throat chakra is used equally for expression and truth. It enables you to take your place in the world.

If your throat chakra is balanced:
You express yourself easily, both in speaking and in writing. You are not frightened to offer your opinion even if you know in advance that it may not be entirely welcome. You are a good speaker and other people listen to and understand you. You know how to impose limits and to say no. Truth is your watchword.

If your throat chakra is unbalanced:
You are unable to express yourself clearly. You prefer to not express your opinion as you are afraid it may anger others. All of these unspoken issues cause a sore throat, a cough and disguised cries for help. You find it hard to say no and you regularly end up doing pointless tasks. You often feel obliged to tell lies.

Dysfunction of the thyroid and toothache are also linked to a lack of energy with this chakra.

To activate your throat chakra:
- Sing
- Draw
- Read out loud
- Keep a diary
- Do some creative writing.

Third eye chakra

Colour: indigo
Physical placement: between the eyebrows
Associated organs: pineal gland, eyes, nervous system
Function: intuition, visualisation
Issues: concentration, clarity

The sixth chakra – *ajna* in Sanskrit – or the third eye chakra, is situated between the eyebrows and is responsible for the head and the pineal gland. It influences intuition and spiritual development. It brings lightness to daily life. It is a very powerful chakra that, if carefully mastered, can take you towards another dimension.

If your third eye chakra is balanced:
You make good decisions and are in a good place at a good time. You have good intuition. You do not ask yourself questions about the meaning of life, which is obvious to you. You have confidence in your future and you concentrate on the present moment. You trust others because your intuition directs you towards reliable people. Your mental capacities like concentration, vigilance and memory are equally well developed.

If your third eye chakra is unbalanced:
You are closed off mentally. You have to plan and calculate everything. Instead of letting go, you are always thinking. You want to assign meaning to everything you do. You are a slave to deadlines and timetables. You do not have faith in your future or in yourself. You do not comprehend your spiritual goal. Your intuition is weak and you are unable to visualise. You suffer frequent headaches.

To activate your third eye chakra:
- Keep a journal of your dreams
- Visualise
- Chant mantras
- Watch the sunset
- Do some gymnastics for your eyes.

Crown chakra

Colour: violet, white or gold
Physical placement: top of the head
Associated organs: cranium, cerebral cortex, endocrine system, pituitary gland
Function: connection to spiritual strength, higher consciousness
Issues: mental confusion, separation from the cosmos

The seventh chakra – *sahasrara* in Sanskrit – or the crown chakra, is situated at the top of the head and is responsible for the head and the pituitary gland.

It is the origin of your life purpose. Its energy allows you to reconnect with God, the cosmos and the universe. This connection manifests itself in your thoughts, your words and your daily acts.

If your crown chakra is balanced:
You feel as though you are guided in life. You feel strong support on your path and you feel worthy of it. You know why you are on the earth and what your purpose is. You have mental clarity and peace, and you are in good health. You are thankful for all you have in your life. Your thoughts, your words and your acts are the manifestation of your inner peace.

If your crown chakra is unbalanced:
You feel lost, confused, abandoned. You are limited by physical reality and your watchword is 'control'. This excessive control provokes a feeling of constant helplessness and makes you unhappy. You fall into a vicious circle that leads to depression. You feel zero spiritual support and have the impression that you are cut off from it. You encounter obstacles that prevent you from advancing or that cause you to abandon your projects. You often get headaches.

To activate your crown chakra:
- Meditate
- Do breathing exercises
- Try fasting
- Pray
- Try yoga inversion postures.

Pranayama, the breath of life

Pranayama in Sanskrit signifies 'mastery of your life force'. In order to control your *prana* – your life force – it is necessary to learn how to breathe. Breathing reflects our emotional state. When it is mastered, it can instil a feeling of general well-being.

When practising yoga, breathing reinforces the depth of each posture to help reconnection with the body. It also helps you to overcome physical and emotional pain on the mat or in life. Ample, deep and fluid respiration calms the spirit, relaxes the body and clears the mind.

Belly breathing

Ventral, or belly, breathing is the most basic kind. It is the breathing of a relaxed person. Babies do it naturally but adults progressively forget it because of stress, a fast pace of life and societal demands. In order to understand this type of breathing, observe a sleeping baby. The belly expands during inhalation and goes in during exhalation. When you are relaxed, your stomach follows this fluid, deep movement. As part of your practice, I suggest you breathe with your stomach most of the time, as ventral breathing improves blood circulation and energy in the lower body, the seat of femininity and female health.

Dynamic breathing

This also comes from the stomach and is very often used in Yoga for Women. It is more rhythmic, like a clock. You breathe in the same manner as with belly breathing by inflating and deflating the stomach, but quicker, in the rhythm of a clock: tick-tock, tick (in), tock (out).

With practice, you can inflate the lower stomach, which is good for femininity and female health. In fact, it boosts the energy that stimulates the ovaries and uterus.

Practise this breathing only in the postures indicated.

Liberating breathing

Liberating breathing is used to relax the body and to liberate negative emotions or spent energy. You simply breathe in deeply through the nose and out through the mouth, while making an 'aah' sound.

When you are active – or hyperactive – your breath speeds up, moves up and builds up in the chest. This is clavicular breathing. Observe the phenomenon in these situations: the more you breathe like this (in more than out), the more stressed you will be.

You can break this habit, and you can exercise breathing in a different way. In order to liberate your breathing, lie down on your back and place one or two hands on your stomach. Relax and feel the melodic movements from your stomach as the air comes in and out.

Let your breathing guide your practice and take plenty of breaks between postures to reconnect with your breathing. Make the most of the life force that fills you as you breathe.

Facial yoga – gestures that do you good

When practising yoga, women tend to favour postures with the body, sometimes forgetting the face. Exposed to the sun, wind and sometimes extreme temperatures, the skin of the face needs a lot of care and attention. A lack of facial muscle exercise manifests itself as wrinkles or a loss of muscle tone. Also, fixed expressions can lead to micro-wrinkles.

Your face is a reflection of your psyche. Your daily emotions and concerns gradually imprint themselves on to your skin and your muscles. The care you take of your face can make all the difference.

Yoga for Women includes various facial yoga exercises aimed to relax and even rejuvenate the face. This is without looking for 'eternal youth', which is incompatible with self-acceptance. The face massages and specific exercises stimulate different parts of the face. The benefits are not limited to the physical – they also influence the emotional state. While you practise, breathe deeply and pay attention to your feelings. Certain exercises may awaken certain unexpected emotions in you. Savour them and carry on. Remember that a smile is the best treatment for your face.

Hasta mudras, gracious gestures

A mudra, which signifies a 'seal', is a precise position of the body, the tongue, the eyes or fingers. The mudra seals the link between our subconscious and ourselves, and between the subconscious and the universe.

In yoga, hand mudras (*hasta mudras*) are the most common. Unlike the body postures that originate in India, hand mudras appear all over the world in different forms. In every religion, including Western ones, there are canonical gestures that correspond to mudras. Outside of the religious spectrum, mudras have found a place in our daily lives: thumbs up or thumbs down (agreement or disagreement), finger raised (to ask permission), the surfer shaka or v-sign, for example.

Mudras can change your emotions and increase your well-being. They act on all levels: physical, emotional, energetic. They are very powerful and are used in many complementary medicines.

In reflexology, each finger and each part of the palm corresponds to a specific organ. By applying pressure to certain points or bending certain fingers, the corresponding organ is stimulated.

In Ayurveda, the traditional Indian healing system, each finger corresponds to an element, and the amount of each element present in our body influences our health. The thumb represents fire, the index finger air, the middle finger ether, the ring finger earth and the little finger water.

In traditional Chinese medicine, many meridians and acupuncture points are found in the fingers and/or the palms of the hands, and can be stimulated by mudras.

In your practice of Yoga for Women, you will use different mudras in order to augment your physical or emotional needs.

Breathe deeply and close your eyes while you perform mudras in order to increase their efficiency.

Mulabandha, the root lock

Bandha is traditionally translated from Sanskrit as 'lock'. There are three locks in the body: one at throat level, one at the centre of the stomach and one at the perineum.

In Yoga for Women, we mostly stimulate the *mulabandha*, the perineum lock, or more precisely, the root chakra. The group of perineal muscles is attached in a diamond shape in front of the pubis, behind the coccyx and two sides of the gluteal muscles. A toned perineum allows good support for the internal organs, prevents a prolapse, prevents faecal and urinary incontinence, helps carry a baby during pregnancy, aids quick recovery after birth, allows you to make the most of sex, and to have a good posture in the back and spine.

On an energetic level, the root lock awakens powerful divine energy, the *kundalini*, that sleeps in the root chakra. When awakened, it rushes along the *sushumna* energy canal and circulates the length of the spine, passing all the chakras and filling the head. Once mastered, following many years of practice, this process leads to fullness.

In certain dynamic yoga postures, this lock is necessary to protect the lower back and to avoid unnecessary pressure on the organs. The basic rule is to tense your perineum upon exhalation before making any effort.

To activate the root lock, tense your perineal muscles as you exhale. The term 'contract' is often used, but is only half right because you have to contract the muscles and *then* tense them. Imagine you have a geisha ball in your vagina and you want to hold it in – it is the same movement. Seal the lock less intensely or avoid it completely during your period.

In your practice of Yoga for Women, you will activate *kundalini* to balance your chakras, stimulate energy circulation in the pelvis and to reconnect with your femininity.

Dhyana, visualisation

Even more complex than the concept of meditation, *dhyana* is a state of mastered concentration. Used at the end of a session to reinforce the *sankalpa*, *dhyana* is visualisation, a creative meditation. It draws on mental strength and the imagination. It allows you to attain a precise goal while staying connected to the present moment, thanks to deep breathing. After working the muscles, the body is ready for the stationary journey into the depths of the subconscious.

The visualisations offered in this book will bring you to the realisation of your projects in accurate imagery. The symbolic images allow you to address different aspects of your psyche and to find solutions to problems. They facilitate our communication with our unconscious, which finds it easier to understand images and symbols than words. By imagining a butterfly in the throat to represent the thyroid, we send a lightweight and healthy message to our subconscious in the endocrine gland.

What is sacred femininity?

Sacred femininity, the expression of pure femininity, manifests itself with a call to feminine nature to reconnect with its core values. Women who awaken this true essence will blossom, be happy and powerful. Conversely, when feminine power fades, self-confidence and self-esteem disappear.

According to Indian sages, the body is the manifestation of the divine in the material world. For centuries, Westerners have rejected and judged – through ignorance – the body, sexual pleasure, the menstrual cycle and old age. In fact, it is in the body – more precisely the pelvis – that a thousand wonders are concealed.

More and more women are answering this deep call. Some want to get over an unhappy past, others simply want to share and enjoy happy moments. All of them are bringing to life the goddess that is dormant inside them, buried by their patriarchal history, family traditions and societal dogmas.

Embark on a discovery of your sacred femininity

On a physical level, the pelvis contains the iliac bones that make the infinity sign with the centre of the pubis, the sacrum that signifies 'sacred' in Latin, the ovaries that give birth to life and the uterus that shelters the foetus until birth.

On an energy level, the pelvis is a bowl that contains the vital energy which we call 'sacred femininity'. It is therefore important for a woman to fill it with fresh energies, by accepting her femininity, her body, her ovaries, her uterus and her periods. The simple act of thinking about them sympathetically and giving them a place in life is beneficial.

Listening to your pelvis can be painful, especially if suffering that has built up over years, generations, centuries has caused an energy heritage in the woman. The most common manifestations of this would be pre-menstrual syndrome (PMS), heavy periods and all gynaecological illnesses.

The menstrual cycle is not just a biological process but equally a spiritual act of nature that is linked to the lunar cycle. Changes in the lunar cycle are reflected – consciously or not – in the different elements of the menstrual cycle.

Understanding these fluctuations brings women closer to their sacred femininity.

Soft approaches, like dance, yoga, breathing exercises and meditation, let you replenish your energy bowl. Yoga for Women makes energy circulate through the pelvis and the whole body to anchor women to their sacred femininity.

Each woman lives the awakening of her sacred femininity differently, but for each one it is obvious. By opening this book you have taken the first step. Follow your path and open yourself up to your sacred femininity!

Two sides of the same coin

In the West, our culture tends towards a system of duality: black and white, good and bad. The notions of feminine and masculine (yin and yang) risk falling into this trap of exclusive classification. They are, however, complementary. Accept the different polarities that are inside of you and direct your attention to your femininity in order to awaken your sacred femininity and find your zest for life.

Feminine and masculine

Evoking psychic bisexuality, Sigmund Freud stated that an individual had two aspects of personality: the softer, enveloping aspect of women and the hard, direct side of men.

This duality shows itself in us through different behaviours in certain situations. A mother is ready to listen with empathy to her grieving child (her female side), but she also knows how to impose limits (her masculine side). A woman can also use her female and male strengths in order to strive to meet life's needs. Nevertheless, women are pushed excessively into masculine energy, notably to stay in control of a situation. The return towards femininity allows you to balance the two extremes and reconnect with female power.

Shakti and Shiva

These two Hindu gods represent the union of the masculine and the feminine. They are often shown as a single person, half-man and half-woman.

Shiva, translated from the Sanskrit as 'good, one who brings luck', is the supreme Hindu god. He symbolises consciousness and masculine energy.

Considered as the god of yoga, meditation and art, he creates, protects and transforms the universe.

Shakti, who signifies 'power', the expression of feminine creativity, is the incarnation of a deity who, through her exhilarating dance, expresses the personality of each human in thought, words and gestures. According to Sally Kempton, Shakti[3] is also the strength that pushes us inevitably towards the evolution of our consciousness, which must take place in order to attain a higher level of consciousness.

The practice of Yoga for Women will help you to awaken this goddess inside you.

Yin and yang

According to Taoist philosophy, notions of yin and yang are complementary and are present everywhere. It is a complex system that goes beyond a simple representation of feminine and masculine.

Yin is black, encourages letting go, stillness, welcome.

Yang, white, takes us in the opposite direction, to reasoned action, control, expression.

Practising Yoga for Women will allow you to go deep into the yin and to express your female nature, which is powerful and soft at the same time.

Earth and sky

Terrestrial energy moves inside the body. This powerful force that comes up from the feet is present in men as well as women. Similarly, celestial forces come down from the sky through the head. In men, celestial energy is more important. In women it is terrestrial energy that is more present. Generally, people in the same family are drawn to and influenced by the mother, who personifies terrestrial strength. She also often holds the psychological responsibility that is linked to the emotional well-being of everyone in the family. This feminine energy is the strength that anchors the woman. So when a woman re-establishes her link with the earth, thanks for example to Yoga for Women, all of the family benefits.

---

3 Author of *Awakening Shakti: The Transformative Power of the Goddesses of Yoga*, Sounds True, 2013.

Mushroom and guitar

A man's energy centre is in the head and manifests itself in action, propulsion and movement. The women's is in the pelvis and appears in acceptance, reception and calmness.

In order to keep their place in society, women often find it necessary to be more masculine in an effort to remain part of the action. Consequently, their energy goes to their head.

The energy portrait of contemporary women would have the form of a mushroom, whereas it should look more like a guitar with energy stored in the pelvis. When the energy makes its way to the pelvis, women are more soothed, calm and anchored. They lose none of their efficiency this way; on the contrary they become relaxed and alert.

The best way to get to this state is to unwind and take some time for yourself.

Ida and pingala

Vital energy is distributed throughout the body through energy channels that are located in the subtle body (*see* page 9). The three principal channels run from their base in the spine and go up, snaking around and crossing over up to the left nostril, *ida*, and the right nostril, *pingala*.

The energy from the *ida* channel is feminine and is calm, relaxed, cold and receptive.

The energy from the *pingala* is masculine and in action, movements of strength, warmth and propulsion.

When these two channels are in balance a third channel, *sushumna*, activates, leading to bliss.

Yoga for Women will help you to harmonise all of your energy channels.

Sun and moon

Ida, the feminine energy channel, is connected to the moon, and *pingala*, the masculine energy, is connected to the sun.

Although both heavenly bodies influence the body and spirit of a woman, the moon is the symbol of femininity. It follows the same cycle as the menstrual cycle (around 28 days) and influences ovulation, menstruation, mood and emotion.

Through gravitational force, the moon reacts powerfully to move the sea with tides. Its influence on the human body, which is more than 60 per cent water, is undeniable. Hormonal changes due to the moon affect our general well-being. The energy centre of the lower abdomen, whose element is water, is also affected by lunar fluctuations and these can be felt as – sometimes unpleasant – sensations.

Discover the four sessions dedicated to lunar phases to help you reconnect with your feminine energy (*see* page 136).

Left and right

Psychology, yoga and traditional Chinese medicine agree on the fact that male–female synergy is present in the body and influences our health and behaviour.

According to yoga, the left side represents the feminine and the right side the masculine. In order to develop female energy, calm, relaxed and receptive, Yoga for Women encourages you to start with left-side postures. In order to resolve physical problems and to stimulate action, warmth and momentum, reverse the positioning.

By being conscious of these elements, you can advance in your practice of Yoga for Women and in your life by releasing tension and spent energy.

How do you practise Yoga for Women?

This is not a book designed for passive reading. I suggest you sit comfortably on your yoga mat or towel to try the postures and exercises I list. Follow the sessions according to your needs, your mood or your desire.

Create a welcoming ambiance by choosing a warm, calm place. Wear comfortable clothes and have a sweater and warm socks handy for calmer sessions. Having your own yoga mat allows you to create your very own ritual for a productive, friendly practice. Get yourself a bolster, roll cushion or a rolled-up blanket to help you with certain gentle postures.

Each session lasts between 15 and 30 minutes; adapt around your own availability and your breathing. For most of the postures I suggest you do them for 5 to 10 breaths, which will be around 1 to 2 minutes. The final relaxation lasts around 5 to 10 minutes and feel free to stretch out if you feel the need.

Ideally, practise dynamic sessions in the morning or during the day, and avoid them in the evening to ensure you sleep well.

It is better to practise on an empty stomach. If you have eaten, ideally wait two hours before a dynamic session and one hour for a gentle session.

Conducting a session

When you have chosen your session, go through each exercise in order to familiarise yourself with the theme. Then, read the instructions for the entire session, in order to stay focused throughout the practice. And when you feel ready, get going.

Each session starts with an intention, the *sankalpa*. If it doesn't suit you completely, feel free to adjust it (*see* page 8).

During the postures, I suggest you nourish certain chakras through breathing. That is to say, you should concentrate on the chakra: imagine a coloured bubble and breathe deeply while keeping this image in your head.

To nourish your ovaries and uterus, concentrate on those organs or simply on the lower abdomen and breathe deeply.

During practice, stay conscious of your body and note the sensations induced by each posture. Do not hesitate to yawn during a gentle session. Yawning is often seen as a sign of boredom, but is in fact a sign of relaxation.

At the end of each session, practise *savasana*, the relaxation posture. This will allow you to integrate the benefits of your practice.

After a gentle session, drink a herbal tea and rest before taking advantage of the effects of your practice.

Try to practise regularly – at least one session per week. This will allow you to stay connected to your sacred femininity.

Observe without judgement the changes that Yoga for Women will bring to your body, your heart and your life.

—

A gentle and safe activity

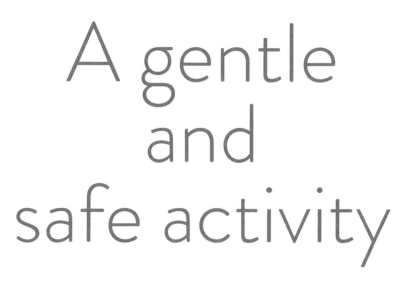

When you practise Yoga for Women you will perform dynamic – yang – postures that are demanding, and relaxed postures – yin – which are mainly done on the floor. Some postures must be carried out with care to avoid the possibility of injury. Others must be avoided during your period or if you are ill. Before starting a session, read the instructions in this section carefully and take note of the recommendations for the appropriate postures.

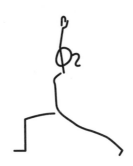

Warrior 1

How to do it

· Stand upright, feet hip-width apart and with your hands on your hips.
· Take a big step back with your left foot so there is roughly 1 metre between your two feet.
· Turn your left foot out. Both feet are well rooted. Try to gradually place your left heel flat on the floor.
· Turn your left hip towards the front to have both hips aligned and bend your right knee. Make sure your knee doesn't go further than your ankle.
· As you exhale, lift your perineum.
· Breathe in and stretch your arms to the sky.
· Keep your arms parallel. If you are comfortable, join your palms together, keeping your shoulders relaxed.
· Look straight ahead of you or look towards your hands without creating too much tension in your neck.

Precautions

The knee of your front leg must not go past your ankle.

Your hips stay facing the front.

Engage your perineum during the posture to stabilise the lower body and protect the lower back. To engage the perineum, remember you must take a deep breath, as if you are trying to hold on to a geisha ball inside your vagina.

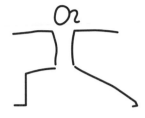

Warrior 2

How to do it

- Stand upright, take a big step back with your left foot so there is roughly 1 metre between your two feet.
- Place your left foot parallel to the edge of the mat to make a right angle with the right foot. Your right heel should be aligned with the middle of your left foot.
- As you exhale, lift your perineum.
- Inhale and lift your arms so they are parallel with the ground. Bend your right knee so that your right thigh is parallel with the ground. Make sure your knee does not go past your ankle.
- Anchor both feet to the ground. Straighten your left leg.
- Align your hips with your legs by lightly pushing your left hip backwards. Keep your shoulders relaxed.
- Look down the length of your right hand.

Precautions

The knee of your front leg must not go past your ankle.

Your hips must be aligned and open, parallel to the sides of your mat.

Engage your perineum during the posture to stabilise the lower body and protect the lower back.

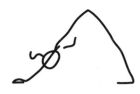

Downward-facing dog

How to do it

- Get on all fours, your hands below your shoulders and your knees open the width of your hips. Hook your toes into the floor.
- As you exhale, straighten your knees by pushing into the floor with your hands and feet.
- Push your coccyx towards the sky keeping your legs slightly bent. Straighten your arms and legs. Relax your head between your arms and keep your ears free of your shoulders.
- Stretch out your back and armpits by gently bending your knees and pushing into the floor with your hands. If you are comfortable, stretch your legs and get your heels flat on the floor.
- Look between your legs.

Precautions

Your back must be straight.

Keep your shoulders clear of your ears.

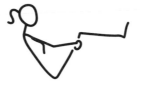

Boat

How to do it

- Sit down, bend your knees and hold the backs of your thighs with your hands.
- Engage your perineum and your abdominal wall.
- As you breathe out, raise your feet one by one to have your shins parallel with the floor. You will naturally tilt backwards. Your back must stay straight.
- If you are comfortable, release your hands and keep your arms parallel to the floor. You can also straighten your legs whilst keeping your back straight. Your feet can be above or at the same level as your head.
- Look at your toes.

Precautions

Tense your perineum and your abdominal wall during the posture in order to protect the lower back.

Make sure you keep your back straight, particularly in the advanced version with straight legs. For that one, push your chest forward and bring your shoulders back.

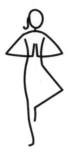

Tree

How to do it

- Stand upright, feet together and place your hands together at chest height.
- Stare at a point in front of you.
- As you exhale, lift your perineum and engage your abdominal wall.
- Shift your weight to the right foot.
- Place your left foot against your right ankle, keeping the toes of your left foot on the floor. If you are comfortable, bring your left foot up to the calf or the inside of your right thigh, above the knee. You may use a hand to help you position your foot.
- Keep your hands together in front of your chest or raise them during inhalation. Keep your shoulders down.

Precautions

Try not to put your foot on your knee.

Look at a fixed point and engage your perineum and abdominal wall during the posture in order to maintain balance.

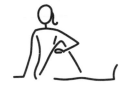

Seated twist

How to do it

- Sit down and stretch out your left leg. Bend your right knee and place your right foot outside your left knee.
- Place your right hand on the floor behind you and your left hand on your right thigh.
- As you breathe in, push yourself up towards the sky.
- As you breathe out, twist a little more by turning your right shoulder to the rear. If you are comfortable, reach under your right knee with your left hand and grasp your right hand behind your back.
- Look over your right shoulder.

Precautions

Start this posture on your right-hand side to stimulate the natural working of the lower intestine.

Keep your back straight by stretching your spine.

After a twist, relax your back with a light turn the other way: do a light twist to the other side without changing the position of your legs.

Not suitable with these conditions

Period – diarrhoea – herniated disc – sciatica – pregnancy

Camel

How to do it

- Kneel down with your knees the same width apart as your hips. Flatten your toes or place your instep on the floor for the advanced version.
- Place your hands at the base of your back, pointing your fingers upwards.
- As you breathe in, stretch your back.
- As you breathe out, lift your perineum and engage your abdominal wall.
- Push your pelvis forward, keeping your head upright. Keep looking towards the space between your eyebrows. If you are comfortable, place one hand on one heel then the other on the other heel and tilt your head backwards.
- After 5 to 10 breaths, as you breathe out, flex your thighs, and engage your perineum and abdominal wall in order to straighten up while gently rolling your head forward.
- Sit down on your heels and put your chest to the floor to relax your back.

Precautions

Engage your perineum, abdominal wall and thighs.

If your neck is tense, keep it straight above your spine and keep looking in front of you.

Not suitable with these conditions

Pregnancy – herniated disc – overactive thyroid

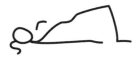

Bridge

How to do it

- Lie on your back, bend your knees with your feet hip width apart.
- Keep your arms straight by your body with your palms facing the floor.
- As you breathe out, engage your perineum and lift your pelvis towards the sky. Keep your knees in line with your hips.
- To increase intensity, squeeze your shoulder blades together, move your arms and interlace your fingers behind your back.
- Keep looking at the space between your eyebrows.

Precautions

Engage your perineum, abdominal wall and thighs.

Keep your knees in line with your hips.

Do not turn your head during this position.

Not suitable with these conditions

Cervical herniated disc – overactive thyroid

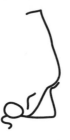

Half-candle

How to do it

- Lie on your back, bend your knees, place your feet on the floor and your arms beside your body.
- Lift your perineum and tense your abdominal wall.
- As you breathe out, raise your hips and bring your knees up to your chest. Bend your elbows and place your hands on each side of your spine to support your lower back.
- As you breathe out, raise your legs to make an angle of roughly 60° between your legs and upper body. Your bodyweight should rest on your shoulders and arms.
- Keep looking at the space between your eyebrows.
- After 5 to 10 breaths, as you breathe out, bend your knees and bring your thighs towards your stomach. Slide your hands towards your buttocks while you gently move your back, bottom and feet to the ground.

Precautions

Engage the perineum and abdominal wall as you go into and leave this posture.

If you have neck pain, place a folded blanket around your upper body. Slide it up to shoulder level, keeping your neck free from the blanket and your head on the floor.

If you have trouble lifting your hips, place a large cushion or rolled-up blanket under your hips and lift your legs up to the sky while keeping your arms beside your body.

Do not turn your head during this posture.

Not suitable with these conditions

Period – diarrhoea – cervical herniated disc – overactive thyroid

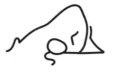

Plough

How to do it

- Lie on your back and bend your knees. Keep the soles of your feet on the floor and your arms the length of your body.
- Lift your perineum and engage your abdominal wall.
- As you breathe out, raise your hips and bring your knees towards your chest. Bend your elbows and place your hands on either side of your spine to support your lower back.
- Let your knees lower towards your face. If you are comfortable, stretch out your legs and put your toes behind your head. For an advanced variation, put your arms flat on the floor beside your body.
- Keep looking at the space between your eyebrows.
- After 5 to 10 breaths, as you breathe out, bend your knees and put your hands on your back again. Bring your thighs towards your stomach and slide your hands towards your buttocks while gently lowering your back, bottom and feet to the floor.

Precautions

Engage the perineum and your abdominal wall when you go in to and out of the posture.

If you have neck pain, place a folded blanket around your upper body. Slide it up to shoulder level, keeping the neck free from the blanket and your head on the floor.

If you have trouble lifting your hips, place a large cushion or rolled-up blanket under your hips, bend your knees and bring them towards your chest while keeping your hands on your shins.

Do not turn your head during this posture.

Not suitable with these conditions

Period – diarrhoea – cervical herniated disc – overactive thyroid

———

The body

Each body has its own story. In my yoga classes I have seen hundreds – thousands – of different bodies, some supple, others stiff, some thin and others heavier; bodies that bear marks of physical or emotional suffering. They are all completely different but at the same time are all united by one common point: their beauty.

Allow your body to tell you its story as you take care of it with the sessions that follow.

And above all, listen to it carefully. It certainly has much to tell you.

Body acceptance

The media forces an image of the 'ideal' woman upon us, with standards to follow that give many women a complex.

We think we are not enough 'this' or too much 'that', and we abuse our bodies with diets, cosmetic and chemical products and – above all – with criticism. To be healthy, our bodies need love and acceptance.

Postures for the sacral chakra and the heart chakra will help you to accept and love your body and your femininity.

🪷 *Write down five parts of your body that you love.*

....

....

....

....

....

Sankalpa

· Sit down with your legs crossed.
· Put your palms together and your fingers upright together in front of your chest. Close your eyes.
· Take some deep breaths and speak your intention in a loud voice: 'I accept my divine, beautiful body.'

Goddess

· Open your arms wide as you breathe in and look up.
· As you breathe out, lower your head and wrap yourself in your arms. Repeat 5 or 6 times.
· The last time, hold yourself in your arms while saying: 'I accept you as you are! You are wonderful!'

Crescent moon

· Get on all fours and place your right foot inside your right
  hand. Anchor to the floor by bending your right knee,
  making sure it does not go past your ankle.
· As you breathe out, lift your perineum.
· As you breathe in, stretch your arms to the ceiling and
  feel your chest open up.
· Keep your shoulders down.
· Look straight in front of you and feed your heart chakra
  for 5 to 10 breaths.
· Do the same on the other side.

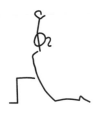

Butterfly

· Sit down, bend your knees and push them towards the
  floor, keeping the soles of your feet together. If you feel
  tension in your knees, place cushions under your thighs to
  support your legs.
· As you breathe out, bend forwards while keeping your hands
  on your feet.
· Feed your sacral chakra for 5 to 10 breaths.
· Straighten your back gently.

Swan

· Bend your left knee more and place your left foot in front of
  your right hip.
· Stretch your right leg out behind you, keeping your
  instep flat on the floor.
· Place your hands each side of your hips and open
  your chest. If you tilt to the left, place a cushion under
  your left buttock.
· Breath deeply, imagining the air comes in and out of your chest
  for 5 to 10 breaths, then do the same on the other side.

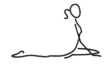

Sleeping swan

- Keeping your right knee bent, bend over forwards and place your forehead on the floor. You can place a cushion under your head.
- Feed your sacral chakra for 5 to 10 breaths.
- Do the same on the other side.

Supine twist

- Lie down on your back with your arms out beside you as a cross.
- Bend your knees towards your chest.
- As you breathe out, move your knees to the left as you turn your head to the right. If you feel tension in your lower back, try placing a cushion under your left leg.
- Feed your sacral chakra for 5 to 10 breaths.
- Do the same on the other side.

Hug

- Stay lying on the floor with your knees bent and together. Feet on the floor, at least hip width apart.
- Hold yourself in your arms. Stay in this position for 1 minute while breathing deeply. Whisper soft words of well-being to yourself.

Magic lotion

- Sit cross-legged and rub the palms of your hands together until you feel heat.
- Place your hands on your face and imagine you are applying a cream made from love and well-being.
- Feed your face and then your hair, neck, shoulders, arms and so on, giving the rest of your body the same attention.

Mudra for loving yourself

- Point your left index finger. Place your right thumb on your left index finder, then wrap the other fingers from your right hand around it.
- Close your eyes and hold the mudra in front of your chest and breathe deeply for 1 minute. Imagine your left index finger is a fragile, beautiful you. Welcome the feelings.

Visualisation

- Keeping your eyes closed, let go of your finger.
- Imagine a light coming from your heart and surrounding you. For 1 minute concentrate on the sensation of feeling this light on your skin.

Savasana

- Lie on your back for the final relaxation, with your legs stretched out in front of you and your arms beside your body with your palms facing upwards.
- Rest for 5 to 10 minutes.

In order to develop your love for your body, stand naked in front of a large mirror. Look carefully at your body with acceptance and kindness. This may seem difficult at first, but with practice, you will find your curves or thinness first acceptable, then adorable.

Mix 70 drops of magnolia essential oil in a bottle with 100ml of vegetable oil. After a shower, carefully put this oil over every part of your body before drying off. Give each part of your body the attention it requires. Then dry yourself carefully with a towel.

Carry a chrysoprase crystal in your pocket to reinforce the link of your body and your femininity. This will make you want to look after yourself more.

Slenderness and tone

A healthy body gives you a zest for life. In order to keep it healthy, a good diet combined with regular sporting activity will support your metabolism, which can weaken during winter, with age, with hormonal changes or weight gain.

Postures that activate the solar plexus chakra, where the fire energy – *Agni* – is stored, are good for stimulating the metabolism, burning toxins and excess calories, as well as for getting rid of deep-rooted fears.

After the session, note down the physical and emotional changes you felt.

....

....

....

....

....

Sankalpa

· Sit down with your legs crossed.
· Put your palms together and your fingers upright together in front of your chest. Close your eyes.
· Take some deep breaths and speak your intention in a loud voice: 'I am dynamic and courageous.'

Warrior 1

- Stand up with your hands on your hips.
- Take a big step backwards with your left leg and turn it outwards.
- Slowly, try to put your left heel on the floor.
- Turn your left hip to the front to keep your hips balanced.
- Bend your right knee but don't let it go further than your ankle.
- Breathe in and stretch your arms up.
- Keep your shoulders down.
- Keep looking straight in front of you and open your solar plexus chakra.
- Do the same on the other side.

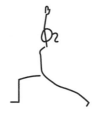

Warrior 2

- Keep your left knee bent.
- Open out your right foot to make a right angle with your left foot.
- Stretch out your arms, parallel with the floor.
- Engage your right leg and look along the length of your left arm.
- Open your solar plexus chakra for 5 to 10 breaths.
- Do the same on the other side.

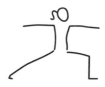

Downward-facing dog

- Get on all fours, and turn your toes under, flat on the floor.
- As you breathe out, push the floor with your hands and toes and lift your pelvis to the ceiling. Keep your knees slightly bent in order to keep your back straight.
- Relax your head, look back between your legs.
- Open your solar plexus chakra for 5 to 10 breaths.

Curled leaf

- Sit on your knees and spread them out.
- Sit back on your heels and keep the tips of your toes together.
- Lower your forehead to the floor, stretch out your back and arms.
- Open your solar plexus chakra for 5 to 10 breaths.

Knee lift

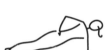

- Lie on your back.
- Bring your right knee up to your chest and grasp it with your hands.
- If you are not on your period, take 5 to 10 dynamic breaths: inflate your stomach as you inhale and relax it as you exhale, to the rhythm of a clock.
- Breathe deeply as you open your solar plexus chakra. Change to the other side.

Half side-plank

- Lie on your left side with your right hand on your hip.
- Place your left forearm at a right angle to the body and lean on it.
- As you breathe out, engage your abdominal wall and lift your perineum.
- Lift your hips from the floor and put your right foot on your left foot.
- If you are comfortable, lift your right hand to the ceiling.
- Open your solar plexus chakra for 5 to 10 breaths.
- Do the same on the other side.

Boat

- Sit down, bend your knees and hold the backs of your thighs with your hands.
- Engage your perineum and your abdominal wall.
- As you breathe out, raise your feet one by one to have your shins parallel with the floor.
- If you are comfortable, release your hands and hold your arms out so they are parallel to the floor.
- Open your solar plexus chakra for 5 to 10 breaths.

Scalp massage

- Sit cross-legged.
- With the tips of your fingers, massage your scalp for 1 minute to stimulate the different reflexology points that are found there.

Shiny skull breath

- Place a hand above your belly button to feel the movement above your belly.
- Breathe out powerfully through your nose, as if you were blowing out a candle. Breathe in naturally.
- Repeat 9 times, imagining you are expelling used energy far from your body.

Visualisation

- Remove your hand.
- Concentrate on your solar plexus and imagine a fire there, burning away your physical and emotional toxins. Feed it each time you breathe in for 1 minute.

Savasana

- Lie on your back for the final relaxation, with your legs stretched out in front of you and your arms beside your body with your palms facing upwards.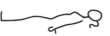
- Rest for 5 to 10 minutes.

Avoid eating for three hours before sleep. Digestive fire slows down at night to prepare the body for rest and toxin evacuation. A late meal risks adding to the toxins and therefore your weight. Also, going to bed just after a meal disturbs your sleep.

- To stimulate digestion, after a meal take 1 drop of mandarin essential oil with a teaspoon of honey.
- For detox, wear a citrine crystal level with your solar plexus chakra.

Youthful bust and arms

The youthfulness of your bust depends on many factors, one of which is the firmness of your pectoral muscles. These are the muscles that are found behind your breasts and give them good structure. Toning your pectoral muscles prevents your bust from sagging. A straight back augments a bust's size visually, as opposed to a curved back, which works in the opposite way.

The postures in this session strengthen the pectoral muscles and improve your posture by opening the heart chakra, which, because of its position in the body, has an influence on the appearance as well as the health of your breasts.

Before this session, look at the position of your bust in a mirror. Look again after the session, and note any differences you see here.

....

....

....

....

Sankalpa

· Sit with your legs crossed.
· Put your palms together and your fingers upright together in front of your chest. Close your eyes.
· Take some deep breaths and speak your intention in a loud voice: 'My chest is beautiful and naturally firm.'

Cow and cat

- Get on all fours with your knees hip width apart. Your feet should be relaxed and your hands should be below your shoulders.
- As you breathe in, bend your back down and look up.
- As you breathe out, arch your back and look between your knees.
- Repeat this movement 5 to 10 times as you open your heart chakra.

Four-limbed staff

- Stay on all fours, engage your abdominal wall and tuck your toes under so that they are flat on the floor.
- As you breathe out, lift your perineum.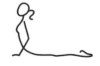
- Bend your arms to make a right angle.
- Stretch your back. Your neck should remain straight at the top of your spine.
- Keep your shoulders down.
- If you are comfortable, lift your knees.
- Take 5 to 10 breaths and take notice of the sensations in the top of your body.

Cobra

- Lie on your front with your feet and legs together.
- Put your hands either side of your ribcage.
- Flatten your feet and engage your perineum.
- As you breathe in, push down with your hands and lift your head, shoulders and chest. Keep your elbows bent and do not lift your shoulders.
- Look in front of you and open your heart chakra for 5 to 10 breaths.
- Put your head back down.

Dolphin

- Get on all fours.
- Put your forearms on the floor, keeping your elbows below your shoulders and your palms flat on the floor.
- As you breathe out, push the floor with your hands and your forearms.
- Straighten your legs as much as you can comfortably.
- Take 5 to 10 breaths while you think about the sensations in your chest and arms.

Cat stretch

- Put your knees on the floor, hip width apart.
- Relax your feet.
- Walk your hands forward to put your forehad on the floor.
- Open your heart chakra for 5 to 10 breaths.

Warrior 1

- Stand up with your hands on your hips.
- Take a big step backwards with your left leg and turn it outwards.
- Slowly, try to put your left heel on the floor.
- Turn your left hip to the front to keep your hips balanced.
- Bend your right knee but don't let it go further than your ankle.
- Breathe in and stretch your arms up.
- Keep your shoulders down.
- Keep looking straight in front of you and open your solar plexus chakra.
- Do the same on the other side.

Open heart

- Sit down and place a bolster or a rolled-up blanket behind your back.
- Lie down slowly on the bolster. If you feel tension in your neck, put a cushion under your head.
- Relax your arms and legs.
- Open your heart chakra for 5 to 10 breaths.

Chest massage

- Sit cross-legged.
- Slide your right palm under your left breast, then the outer side, below the chest and up to the left collarbone.
- With your left hand, slide from the outside of your left breast to the sternum, going under and between your breasts.
- Repeat the movement 10 times and then do the same thing on the other breast starting with the left hand.

Chest mudra

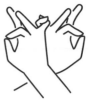

- Cross your fists and link your little fingers.
- Join the tips of the thumb and index fingers on both hands. The other two fingers stay straight.
- Close your eyes and hold your hands in front of your chest.
- Breath deeply as you imagine the air going in and out of your chest for 1 minute.

Visualisation

- Relax your hands and keep your eyes closed.
- Imagine your breasts as two beautiful flowers. Feed the flowers for 1 minute. Receive the sensations.

Savasana

- Lie on your back for the final relaxation, with your legs stretched out in front of you and your arms beside your body with your palms facing upwards.
- Rest for 5 to 10 minutes.

To tone up the skin of your breasts and make it more supple, pass an ice cube made from a base of chamomile or calendula tisane over them. Draw in a spiral starting from the outside and ending around the nipples.

After the ice massage, apply a mixture of 10 to 15 drops of pomegranate essential oil and 30ml of vegetable oil to your breasts.

To make energy circulate in your breasts, wear a malachite pendant at heart level or in the middle of your chest.

Light legs

A sensation of heaviness in the legs may be caused by sitting or standing for a long time, hormonal disruption, venous insufficiency, age, being overweight etc.

The postures in this session will activate the root chakra. They help strengthen muscles in the legs and improve blood and energy circulation. If you frequently have the feeling of heavy legs, make sure you look after yourself properly and seek medical help.

🪷 *On a scale of 0 to 10 (0 being the lightest and 10 the heaviest), rate the sensation of heaviness in your legs. Then do the same when you have finished the session. Note down the differences here.*

....

....

....

....

....

Sankalpa

· Sit down with your legs crossed.
· Put your palms together and your fingers upright together in front of your chest. Close your eyes.
· Take some deep breaths and speak your intention in a loud voice: 'I let used energy flow out.'

Triangle

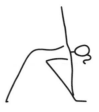

- Stand up straight.
- Take a big step back with your right foot and turn it out so it makes a right angle with your left foot.
- Straighten your arms to shoulder height, keeping them parallel to the floor.
- As you breathe out, lift your perineum and keep your hips forward.
- Bend over to the left and put your left hand on your shin.
- Stretch your right hand to the ceiling.
- Open your root chakra for 5 to 10 breaths.
- Do the same on the other side.

Chair

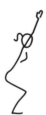

- Place your legs and feet together.
- As you breathe in, bend your knees as if you were going to sit. Raise your arms at the same time and look between your hands.
- Open your root chakra for 5 to 10 breaths.

Tiger

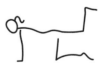

- Get on all fours with your knees hip width apart. Your feet should be flat and your hands should be below your shoulders.
- As you breathe in, lift your left leg up and bend your back gently.
- As you breathe out, bring the knee to the forehead while arching your back. Repeat 4 times on each side and concentrate on the sensations in your back and your legs.

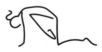

Seed

- Lie on your back.
- Bring your legs to your chest and wrap your arms around them.
- If you are not on your period, take 5 to 10 dynamic breaths: inflate your stomach as you inhale and relax it as you exhale, to the rhythm of a clock.
- Otherwise, breathe deeply and open your sacral chakra.

Bridge

- Bend your knees with your feet hip width apart.
- Keep your arms straight by your body with your palms facing downwards.
- Breathe out, lift your perineum and push your pelvis upwards.
- Open your root chakra for 5 to 10 breaths.

Caterpillar

- Sit down with your legs out straight in front of you.
- As you breathe out, bring your upper body forwards to your legs. Keep your legs and arms relaxed.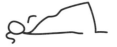
- Open your root chakra for 5 to 10 breaths.

Feet up the wall

- Lie on your back so you can raise your legs upwards.
- Use your heels and elbows to get your bottom right up to the wall.
- Relax your arms along the sides of your body.
- Open your root chakra for 5 to 10 breaths.

Foot massage

- Sit cross-legged.
- Slide the knuckles of one hand along the sole of one foot for 1 minute.
- Repeat the massage on the other foot.

Kali mudra

- Interlace your fingers, apart from your two index fingers which you point together.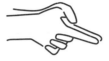
- Cross your left thumb over your right.
- Place the mudra over your shins, pointing the index fingers towards the floor.
- Close your eyes and imagine that your worries and tiredness from the day are leaving through your index fingers in a cloud of dark-coloured smoke. Little by little the colour becomes clearer. You should feel lighter.
- Hold the mudra while breathing deeply for 1 minute.
- Thank the earth for transforming the used energy into positive energy.

Visualisation

- Keeping your eyes closed, relax your hands. Meditate for 1 minute on the lightness that is now inside you.

Savasana

- Lie on your back for the final relaxation, with your legs stretched out in front of you and your arms beside your body with your palms facing upwards.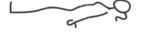
- Rest for 5 to 10 minutes.

Take care of your legs every evening. Shower your legs in warm water at first, then finish off with a jet of cold. Do this 3 or 4 times, always ending with cold water. This shower will help reinforce the blood vessel walls and improve circulation of blood in the legs.

To combat heaviness, massage your arches and legs from bottom to top, with a mixture of 5 drops of patchouli oil in 1 teaspoon of vegetable oil.

Carry a heliotrope or a red pomegranate in your pocket (close to your root chakra), to improve blood circulation in your legs.

—

The hormonal system

Female well-being depends largely on the state of our endocrine and reproductive systems. They are both linked to our emotions and our beliefs regarding femininity. Female maladies often reflect a resistance to the acceptance of femininity. Gentleness and acceptance are the principal ingredients for our relationship with sacred femininity.

Be patient and tolerant. Your being (body and spirit) is a complex, sophisticated structure that needs time to perform certain procedures (pregnancy is the perfect example) or to cleanse a dysfunction or imbalance.

Grant yourself a moment of ease and softness with these sessions and learn to look after yourself well every day.

Active oestrogen phase

Reminder: do not perform this session until after your period.

The physical and emotional state of a woman depends largely on her menstrual cycle.

You will notice the differences more if you follow the two phases of your period. The first phase is the oestrogen phase which starts on the first day of your period and lasts two weeks (based on a 28-day menstrual cycle).

It is the time when the body and morale are at their best. Dynamic practice is therefore to be welcomed. Yang postures, linked to your root chakra and your solar plexus chakra, will do you a lot of good.

🪷 *Before the session, note down the projects that you want to get underway in the next two weeks.*

....

....

....

....

....

Sankalpa

- Sit down with your legs crossed.
- Put your palms together and your fingers upright together in front of your chest. Close your eyes.
- Take some deep breaths and speak your intention in a loud voice: 'I am powerful and focused.'

Warrior 2

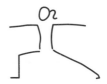

- Stand up. Take a big step back with your left foot and turn it out to make a right angle with the right foot.
- Bend your right knee but do not let it go past your ankle.
- Lift your arms so they are parallel with the floor.
- Tense your right leg and look along the length of your right arm.
- Open your solar plexus chakra for 5 to 10 breaths.
- Do the same on the other side.

Chair

- Come back to the front of the mat and place your legs and feet together.
- As you breathe in, bend your knees as if you were going to sit.
- Raise your arms at the same time and look between your hands.
- Open your root chakra for 5 to 10 breaths.

Downward-facing dog

- Get on all fours, and hook your toes to the floor.
- As you breathe out, push the floor with your hands and toes and lift your pelvis to the ceiling. Keep your knees slightly bent in order to keep your back straight.
- Relax your head, look back between your legs.
- Open your solar plexus chakra for 5 to 10 breaths.

Four-limbed staff

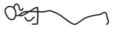

- Put your knees back on the floor, engage your abdominal wall and tuck your toes under so that they are flat on the floor.
- As you breathe out, lift your perineum.
- Bend your arms to make a right angle, keeping your knees on the floor.
- Stretch your back.
- Keep your shoulders down. Your neck should remain straight at the top of your spine.
- If you are comfortable, lift your knees.
- Take 5 to 10 breaths and take notice of the sensations in the top of your body.

Boat

- Sit down, bend your knees and hold the backs of your thighs with your hands.
- Tense your perineum and your abdominal wall.
- As you breathe out, raise your feet one by one to have your shins parallel with the floor. If you are comfortable, release your hands and hold your arms out.
- Open your solar plexus chakra for 5 to 10 breaths.

Bridge

- Lie on your back.
- Bend your knees with your feet hip width apart.
- Keep your arms straight by your body with your palms facing downwards.
- Breathe out, lift your perineum and push your pelvis upwards.
- Take 5 to 10 dynamic breaths: inflate your stomach as you inhale and relax it as you exhale, to the rhythm of a clock.

Half-candle

- Lie on your back, bend your knees, place your feet on the floor and your arms beside your body.
- Lift your hips and bring your knees up to your chest.
- Bend your elbows and place your hands on each side of your spine to support your lower back.
- As you breathe out, raise your legs to make an angle of roughly 60° between your legs and upper body. Your bodyweight should rest on your shoulders and arms.
- After 5 to 10 breaths, as you breathe out, bend your knees and bring your thighs towards your stomach.
- Slide your hands towards your buttocks while you gently move your back, bottom and feet to the ground.

Neck strengthening

· Sit cross-legged.
· Place a fist under your chin.
· Breathe in and then, as you breathe out, create resistance between the two.
· Repeat 9 times.

Akash mudra

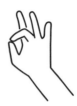

· Link the tips of your middle fingers and your thumbs; your other fingers should point upwards.
· Hold the mudra at shoulder level.
· Close your eyes and breathe deeply for 1 minute.
· Feel the power building in you, filling your entire body.

Visualisation

· Place your hands on your knees.
· Think of a project that means something to you and that you find difficult. Take a few breaths. Imagine you are dealing with this project step by step. Take notice of the satisfaction you feel at the final step. Imagine the final result and the emotions this brings up in you.

Savasana

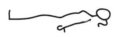

· Lie on your back for the final relaxation, with your legs stretched out in front of you and your arms beside your body with your palms facing upwards.
· Rest for 5 to 10 minutes.

During the oestrogen phase you have a lot of energy. Make the most of this time to start new projects. Take on the thing you usually postpone. Open up to people and make new friends. Put yourself where the action is.

Before this session, or daily if you wish, put a drop of bay tree essential oil on the base of your neck to give you more courage.

Wear a garnet stone during the oestrogen phase to boost your positive energy.

Passive progesterone phase

From the fifteenth day of your cycle (based on a 28-day menstrual cycle) progesterone, the most important hormone for pregnancy, takes over. This harder phase lasts two weeks and ends with your period. It is a time to calm down. It is the autumn of the body and spirit. You may notice mood swings and find yourself more tired than usual. The key to the progesterone phase is: 'Slow down!'

During this phase we do more lunar, 'feminine' postures (sitting or lying, or with gentle stretching). Practise your yoga calmly for your well-being.

❀ Write down two or three ways you will pamper yourself over the two weeks.

....

....

....

....

....

Sankalpa

- Sit down with your legs crossed.
- Put your palms together and your fingers upright together in front of your chest. Close your eyes.
- Take some deep breaths and speak your intention in a loud voice: 'I will take care of myself.'

Torso rotation

- Sit cross-legged, place your hands on your thighs or knees.
- Rotate your body from the pelvis up. Begin with an anti-clockwise rotation and then rotate clockwise.
- Open your root chakra for 5 to 10 breaths in each direction.

Garland

- Crouch down with your feet flat on the floor. If you cannot do this, place a folded blanket beneath your heels.
- Push your knees out and lean your body gently forward.
- Place your palms together in front of your chest.
- Stretch out your back by pushing your elbows against your knees.

Crescent moon

- Get on all fours and place your right foot inside your right hand. Anchor to the floor by bending your right knee, making sure it does not go past your ankle.
- As you breathe out, lift your perineum.
- As you breathe in, stretch your arms to the ceiling and feel your chest open up.
- Keep your shoulders down.
- Look straight in front of you and open your heart chakra for 5 to 10 breaths.
- Do the same on the other side.

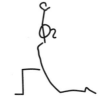

Triskelion

- Sit down.
- Bend your left leg so your left foot points inside.
- Bend your right leg to the outside so your right foot is behind you.
- Bend slowly over your left knee and bring your forehead to the floor.
- Open your sacral chakra for 5 to 10 breaths.
- Do the same on the other side.

Supported bridge

- Lie on your back.
- Bend your knees.
- Gently lift your hips and slide a cushion or bolster underneath.
- Widen the space between your feet and bring your knees together.
- Put your hands on your stomach or beside your body.
- Channel energy to your ovaries and your uterus for 5 to 10 breaths.

Happy baby

- Remove the cushion but stay on your back.
- Bring your knees up to your chest.
- Hold the tips of your toes with your hands.
- Push your knees downwards, keeping your sacrum and head on the floor.
- Open your sacral chakra for 5 to 10 breaths.

Supine twist

- Place your arms out beside you in a cross.
- Bend your knees towards your chest.
- As you breathe out, move your knees to the left as you turn your head to the right. If you feel tension in your lower back, try placing a cushion under your left leg.
- Breathe deeply for 1 minute, concentrating on your right side. Relax.
- Do the same on the other side.

Forehead massage

· Sit cross-legged. With your fist, massage your forehead with horizontal movements for 1 minute.

Moon breathing

· Keep your right hand near your face and relax your right hand.
· Block your right nostril with your right thumb and close your eyes.
· Take 5 to 10 deep breaths through your left nostril.
· Visualise the clear, brilliant light that is entering your left nostril and filling your pelvic region.

Visualisation

· Keeping your eyes closed, release your right hand. Imagine the light overflowing within you.
· Feel the soothing effects of the light.

Savasana

· Lie on your back for the final relaxation, with your legs stretched out in front of you and your arms beside your body with your palms facing upwards.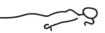
· Rest for 5 to 10 minutes.

During the progesterone phase we lack energy. Slow down: clear your diary, do less and rest more. Plan some 'you time'. Make the most of this time to meditate, keep a private diary and take stock.

 To help you relax even more, spray lavender essential oil around you.

Carry a blue moonstone with you during the progesterone phase to help you reconnect with yourself.

Premenstrual syndrome

Premenstrual syndrome (PMS) is an uncomfortable state that occurs one or two weeks before your period. It includes physical and emotional symptoms such as headaches, sore breasts, mood swings, a heavy feeling in the lower abdomen, or swelling.

The body is sending us a message to adapt our lifestyle during this time.

Take time to listen to and connect with your root chakra and sacral chakra. Gentle postures which stimulate circulation in the lower abdomen are beneficial during this time.

Write down any symptoms you get before your period.

....

....

....

....

....

Sankalpa

- Sit down with your legs crossed.
- Put your palms together and your fingers upright together in front of your chest. Close your eyes.
- Take some deep breaths and speak your intention in a loud voice: 'I am free to be myself.'

Salamander

- Lie on your front with your hands under your face.
- Relax your hips, legs and feet.
- Open your sacral chakra for 5 to 10 breaths.

Curled leaf

- Get up, bend your knees and sit on your heels.
- Keep the tips of your toes together.
- Lower your forehead to the floor, stretch out your back and arms.
- Continue to open your sacral chakra for 5 to 10 breaths.

Seated twist

- Sit down with your legs out in front of you.
- Bend your right knee and place your right foot outside your left knee.
- Place your right hand on the floor behind you and your left hand on your right hip.
- As you breathe in, push yourself upwards.
- As you breathe out, turn your right shoulder behind you.
- Look over your right shoulder.
- Open your solar plexus chakra for 5 to 10 breaths.
- Repeat on the other side.

Seed

- Lie on your back.
- Bring your legs to your chest and wrap your arms around them.
- Open your solar plexus chakra for 5 to 10 breaths.

False inhalation

- Put your feet on the floor and bend your knees.
- Widen your feet but keep your knees touching.
- Put your hands above your stomach.
- Breathe deeply and at the end of your outward breath hold it. Still holding your breath, open up your ribcage as if you were breathing in. Feel your stomach move. Hold for 4 to 6 seconds then breathe in.
- Repeat twice.

Butterfly

- Sit down, bend your knees and push them towards the floor, keeping the soles of your feet together. If you feel tension in the knees, place cushions under your thighs to support your legs.
- As you breathe out, bend forwards while keeping your hands on your feet.
- Nourish your ovaries and your uterus for 5 or 10 breaths.
- Straighten your back gently.

Supine twist

- Lie down.
- Bring your arms out beside you as a cross.
- Bend your knees towards your chest.
- As you breathe out, move your knees to the left as you turn your head to the right. If you feel tension in your lower back, try placing a cushion under your left leg.
- Breathe deeply for 1 minute while you concentrate on your right side. Relax.
- Do the same on the other side.

Ear massage

- Sit cross-legged.
- Rub your palms together until you feel heat.
- Close your eyes.
- Cup your hands over your ears. Very gently rotate 3 or 4 times towards the front and 3 or 4 times to the back.
- Say to yourself: 'I love you. You are perfect.'

Stomach massage

· Rub your palms again.

· With one hand circle your stomach 10 times clockwise (start below the stomach and end at the belly button).

Visualisation

· Put your hands on your knees.

· Close your eyes and concentrate on your lower body. Imagine a line that goes from your coccyx to the centre of the earth. For 1 minute think of all the uncomfortable feelings and negative emotions that descend along this line into the earth to become light.

Savasana

· Lie on your back for the final relaxation, with your legs stretched out in front of you and your arms beside your body with your palms facing upwards.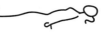

· Rest for 5 to 10 minutes.

To relieve pre-menstrual symptoms, opt for a healthy diet during the second part of your cycle. Eat more wholegrains and vegetables (especially green vegetables). Avoid sugary snacks, and choose instead fruit and dark chocolate, which is rich in magnesium.

The week before your period, massage yourself around the lower abdomen twice a day with a mixture of 1 drop of rosemary verbenone in 4 drops of vegetable oil. This will help to relieve the symptoms. (Do not use if you have been diagnosed with high progesterone or in cases of hormone-sensitive cancer.)

Wear a green opal, either carried in your pocket or worn on your lower abdomen, to balance your hormones.

Menstruation and period pains

For our ancestors, periods were an expression of our sacred femininity. These days they are simply an inconvenience.

Non-acceptance of this natural process can cause uncomfortable feelings during your period. Instead of rejecting it, consider it as a physical and emotional clearout. It is a time for sorting, forgiving and letting go.

Poses for opening your hips help you to open your root chakra and sacral chakra, as well as to relax the lower abdominal muscles to lessen painful feelings.

🪷 *On a scale of 0 to 10 (0 being lightest and 10 the most painful), rate the pain and discomfort you experience. Do the same thing after your yoga session. Note down the changes.*

....

....

....

....

....

Sankalpa

· Sit down with your legs crossed.
· Put your palms together and your fingers upright together in front of your chest. Close your eyes.
· Take some deep breaths and speak your intention in a loud voice: 'I accept, I forgive, I let go.'

Torso rotation

- Sit cross-legged, place your hands on your thighs or knees.
- Rotate your body from the pelvis up. Begin with anti-clockwise rotations and then rotate clockwise.
- Open your root chakra for 5 to 10 breaths in each direction.

Liberating breath

- Place your hands on your lower abdomen and make a triangle with your index fingers and thumbs.
- Inhale deeply through your nose and make yourself bigger.
- Breathe out of your mouth while making an 'aaah' sound and imagining you are breathing out used energy.

Garland

- Crouch down with your feet flat on the floor. If you cannot do this, place a folded blanket beneath your heels.
- Push your knees out and lean your body gently forward.
- Place your palms together in front of your chest.
- Stretch out your back by pushing your elbows against your knees.
- Take 5 to 10 liberating breaths.

Dragonfly

- Sit down with your legs apart in front of you.
- Place a cushion in front of you to go beneath your upper body.
- As you breathe out, lean gently forward. Your back should be relaxed and curved.
- Open your sacral chakra for 5 to 10 breaths.

Reclining butterfly

- Lie on your back.
- Bend your knees and open them outwards, keeping the soles of your feet together.
- Place your hands beside your body or on your lower belly in a triangle mudra: only your thumbs and index fingers touch to form a triangle. The other fingers are straight.
- Channel energy to your ovaries and your uterus for 5 to 10 breaths.

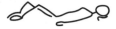

Open heart

- Sit down and place a bolster or a rolled-up blanket at the base of your spine.
- Lie down slowly along the bolster. If you feel tension in your neck, put a cushion under your head.
- Relax your arms and legs.
- Take 5 to 10 liberating breaths.

Foetus

- Bend your knees and roll over to your right side.
- Put your arms under your head.
- Feed your heart chakra for 5 to 10 breaths.

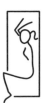

Trapezius massage

- Sit cross-legged.
- Rub the palms of your hands together until you feel heat.
- Put your left hand over your right trapezius muscle at the top of your shoulder, where it meets your neck.
- Slide your hand towards your left collarbone, pressing down firmly.
- Do the same thing with your right hand on your left trapezius muscle. Imagine that you are getting rid of emotional burdens.

Period mudra

· Place the tips of your ring fingers and little fingers on the tips of your thumbs.
· Join both sets of fingers together. The index and middle fingers stay pointing out straight.
· Close your eyes and hold the mudra at the level of your lower abdomen while breathing deeply for 1 minute. Imagine a beautiful, shiny red lotus at the level of your coccyx.
· Feed it during each breath and feel the sensations it brings.

Visualisation

· Place your hands on your knees.
· Concentrate on the red lotus and imagine its stem going into the ground. For 1 minute think of all the uncomfortable feelings and negative emotions that are going down the stem into the earth to become light.

Savasana

· Lie on your back for the final relaxation, with your legs stretched out in front of you and your arms beside your body with your palms facing upwards.
· Rest for 5 to 10 minutes.

Try to make your period more comfortable by looking after yourself. Eat well, exercise and stay warm. Relax as often as you can to reduce stress, which is often the main cause of pain.

To relieve pain, massage your lower abdomen with a mixture of 5 drops of clove oil in 1 teaspoon of vegetable oil. Repeat this massage 4 or 5 times, leaving a minimum of 20 minutes between each massage.

Place two warm chrysocolla crystals on each ovary or carry them in your pockets to relieve pain.

Libido

For a woman, the libido is the barometer of physical and emotional health and her connection to her femininity.

Factors affecting desire are numerous: illness, hormonal changes (especially during the menopause), emotional shock, tiredness, stress etc.

If you think there is a medical reason for a diminishing libido, consult your doctor. Otherwise, use these postures to stimulate your root chakra and your sacral chakra, and rediscover your desire.

🪷 *After the session, think about the sensations in your lower body. Note them down here.*

....

....

....

....

Sankalpa

· Sit down with your legs crossed.
· Put your palms together and your fingers upright together in front of your chest. Close your eyes.
· Take some deep breaths and speak your intention in a loud voice: 'I enjoy life's pleasures.'

Inner perception

· Lie on your back with your legs straight and relaxed.
· Place your hands on your ovaries: thumbs and index fingers touching to form a triangle.
· Breathe in deeply and inflate your stomach fully.
· As you breathe out, deflate it.
· Open your sacral chakra for 10 to 15 breaths.

Supported bridge

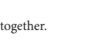

- Bend your knees.
- Gently lift your hips and slide a cushion or bolster underneath.
- Widen the space between your feet and bring your knees together.
- Put your hands on your stomach or beside your body.
- Breathe naturally, lifting and relaxing your perineum dynamically 21 times.

Stretch twist

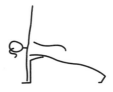

- Get on all fours.
- Put your right foot inside your right hand.
- Turn out the toes on your left foot to aid stability.
- Put your left hand on the floor inside your left foot and raise your right hand upwards.
- Stretch both hands as you push on the floor. If you are comfortable, tense your left leg.
- Look in front of you, upwards.
- If it is not your period, take 5 to 10 dynamic breaths: inflate your stomach as you inhale and relax it as you exhale, to the rhythm of a clock.
- Change to the other knee.

Pelvic rotation

- Stand up with your feet hip width apart. Put your hands on your hips.
- Make a figure of eight with your hips.
- Do the movement 10 times one way, then 10 times the other.

Crescent moon

- Get on all fours and place your right foot inside your right hand. Anchor to the floor by bending your right knee, making sure it does not go past your ankle.
- As you breathe out, lift your perineum.
- As you breathe in, stretch your arms to the ceiling and feel your chest open up.
- Keep your shoulders down.
- Look straight in front of you and feed your sacral chakra for 5 to 10 breaths.
- Do the same on the other side.

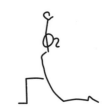

Knee lift

- Lie on your back.
- Bring your right knee up to your chest and grasp it with your hands.
- If you are not on your period, take 5 to 10 dynamic breaths: inflate your stomach as you inhale and relax it as you exhale, to the rhythm of a clock.
- Otherwise, breathe deeply as you open your sacral chakra. Change to the other side.

Reclining butterfly with support

- Sit down and place a bolster or rolled-up blanket at the base of your spine.
- Lie slowly back along the bolster. If you feel tension in the neck, put a cushion under your head.
- Bend your knees and open them outwards, keeping the soles of your feet together.
- Channel energy to your sacral chakra for 5 to 10 breaths.

Bee breathing

- Sit cross-legged.
- Breathe in through the nose and out through the mouth, allowing your lips to vibrate. Do this 4 times.
- Feel the looseness of your cheeks and lips.

Shakti mudra

- Make two fists, keeping your thumbs inside.
- Straighten both ring fingers and little fingers so the tips touch each other. The knuckles of both index and middle fingers should touch.
- Close your eyes and hold the mudra for 1 minute in front of your lower abdomen. The ring fingers and little fingers should point outwards.
- Imagine Shakti, the feminine Indian goddess, looking at you with love and goodwill. Welcome the sensations.

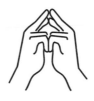

Visualisation

- Relax your hands onto your hips.
- Concentrate on your lower abdomen and imagine a beautiful orange lotus there. Feed it by breathing for 1 minute. Imagine the colour becoming more vivid and bright with each breath.

Savasana

- Lie on your back for the final relaxation, with your legs stretched out in front of you and your arms beside your body with your palms facing upwards.
- Rest for 5 to 10 minutes.

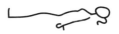

Do some activities that stimulate your sacral chakra: hot, bubbly baths, massages, walks in nature, listening to music, looking at works of art.

To stimulate sexual desire, massage your lower abdomen and lower back with a mixture of 2 to 3 drops of ginger essential oil in 1 teaspoon of vegetable oil.

Use a green jade geisha ball from China to tone your perineum and make more of your sexuality.

Antenatal

During pregnancy, a woman's body becomes a temple that shelters a whole new life. For the baby, it is a house where it is looked after, fed and protected for nine months. It is in the child's and mother's best interests that this house is made as comfortable as possible.

Each pregnancy is different. Nevertheless, the process is the same: the foetus and the liquids surrounding it take up more and more room.
The perineum is always more compressed and the centre of gravity moves. It is common to experience back pain.

The postures in this session restore balance, spine mobility and tone the perineum.

🪷 *Note down your physical and emotional feelings before and after the session.*

....

....

....

....

....

Sankalpa

· Sit down with your legs crossed.
· Put your palms together and your fingers upright together in front of your chest. Close your eyes.
· Take some deep breaths and speak your intention in a loud voice: 'I trust my body and the universe.'

Curled leaf

- Sit on your knees and spread them out.
- Sit back on your heels and keep the tips of your toes together.
- Lower your forehead to the floor, stretch out your back and arms.
- Open your solar plexus chakra for 5 to 10 breaths.

Downward-facing dog

- Get on all fours, and curl your toes into the floor.
- As you breathe out, push the floor with your hands and toes and lift your pelvis to the ceiling. Keep your knees slightly bent in order to keep your back straight.
- Relax your head, look back between your legs.
- Take 5 to 10 breaths, lifting up your perineum each time you breathe out.

Warrior 2

- As you breathe out, walk forward on your hands.
- Roll up your back, vertebra by vertebra, keeping your knees bent.
- Take a big step backwards with your left foot and turn it out so that it makes a right angle with your right foot.
- Lift your arms so they are parallel with the floor.
- Bend your right knee and don't let it go past your right shin.
- Tense your left leg and look along your right arm.
- Take 5 to 10 breaths, lifting up your perineum each time you breathe out.
- Do the same on the other side.

Tree

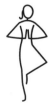

- Put your palms together in front of your chest and put your weight on your right foot.
- As you breathe out, lift your perineum and engage your abdominal wall.
- Place your left foot against your right calf.
- Open your root chakra for 5 to 10 breaths.
- Do the same on the other side.

Reclining butterfly with support

- Sit down and place a bolster or rolled-up blanket at the base of your spine.
- Lie slowly back along the bolster. If you feel tension in the neck, put a cushion under your head.
- Bend your knees and open them outwards, keeping the soles of your feet together.
- Put your hands beside your body or on your stomach and send positive messages to your baby for 5 to 10 breaths.
- Put your legs together and roll onto your side to get out of this posture.

Bridge

- Lie on your back.
- Bend your knees with your feet hip width apart.
- Keep your arms straight by your body with your palms facing downwards.
- Breathe out, lift your perineum and push your pelvis upwards.
- Take 5 to 10 breaths in this position, lifting up your perineum each time you breathe out.
- Lower your pelvis to the floor.

Feet up the wall

- Lie on your back so you can raise your legs upwards.
- Use your heels and elbows to get your bottom right up to the wall.
- Relax your arms along the sides of your body.
- Open your root chakra for 10 to 15 breaths.

Lymphatic massage

- Sit down cross-legged.
- Raise up your left arm and cover your left hand with your right hand.
- Gently draw the right hand towards the armpit, along the side of the left breast and then to the middle of your breastbone.
- Repeat twice and then change sides.

- Massage again starting at the toes then the front and rear of the legs towards the groin, finishing at your hips.
- Repeat twice.

Mudra for calm

- Place your hands on your knees.
- Put your index fingers on the base of the thumbs of both hands. The thumbs go round the index fingers.
- Close your eyes and breathe deeply for 1 minute as you welcome feelings of inner peace.

Visualisation

- Relax your hands and put them on your belly.
- Imagine your baby there, happy and safe inside you. For 1 minute send them messages of peace, love and calmness.

Savasana

- Lie on your back for the final relaxation, with your legs stretched out in front of you and your arms beside your body with your palms facing upwards.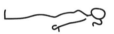
- Rest for 5 to 10 minutes. If you are very heavily pregnant and you are not comfortable on your back, rest in the foetal position (*see* page 74) on your left side.

According to scientists, hearing is the first sense a baby develops. Speak to your baby every day; make them listen to music, read stories and poems loudly to them. Nourish them with love.

Avoid essential oils during pregnancy.

Wear a blue or clear moonstone during your pregnancy.

Post-pregnancy

The joy of childbirth is unique. You finally meet your child. But the reality is not always joyful. Physical and hormonal changes, an emptiness inside felt after childbirth, and attention concentrated upon the child can bring feelings of sadness, emptiness and abandonment.

The postures in this session help you to recover physically and emotionally. You can start these six to eight weeks after giving birth, and until you feel fine.

🪷 *Do this session two or three (or more) times per week and note down the physical and emotional changes you feel.*

....

....

....

....

Sankalpa

· Sit down with your legs crossed.
· Put your palms together and your fingers upright together in front of your chest. Close your eyes.
· Take some deep breaths and speak your intention in a loud voice: 'I feed myself with love to share it with those I love.'

False inhalation

· Lie on your back.
· Bend your knees, widen your feet but keep your knees together. Put your hands on your upper chest.
· Breathe deeply and at the end of your outward breath, hold it. Still holding your breath, open up your ribcage as if you were breathing in. Feel your stomach move. Hold for 4 to 6 seconds then breathe in.

Bridge

· Bend your knees with your feet hip width apart.
· Keep your arms straight by your body with your palms facing downwards.
· Breathe out, lift your pelvis up, hold your breath and engage your perineum.
· As you breathe out, release the perineum and bring your pelvis back to the floor.
· Repeat the movement 9 times.

Aeroplane

· Stand upright with the weight of your body on your right foot and straighten your arms.
· As you breathe out, lift your perineum and engage your abdominal wall. Lean over frontwards by lifting your left leg until your body and left leg are both parallel with the floor.
· Take 5 to 10 breaths as you maintain balance.
· Do the same on the other side.

Triangle

· Take a big step back with your right foot and turn it out to make a right angle with your left foot.
· Straighten your arms to shoulder height, keeping them parallel to the floor.
· As you breathe out, lift your perineum and keep your hips forward as you bend over to the left.
· Put your left hand on your shin or your left foot.
· Stretch your right hand to the ceiling.
· As you breathe out, lift your perineum and suck in your stomach.
· As you breathe in, let them go.
· Take 5 to 10 breaths like this.
· Do the same on the other side.

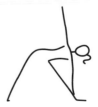

Half side-plank

- Lie on your left side with your right hand on your hip.
- Place your left forearm at a right angle to the body and lean on it.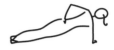
- As you breathe out, engage your abdominal wall and lift your perineum.
- Lift your hips from the floor and put your right foot on your left foot.
- If you are comfortable, lift your right hand to the ceiling.
- Open your solar plexus chakra for 5 to 10 breaths.
- Do the same on the other side.

Half-candle

- Lie on your back.
- Bend your knees and lie your arms beside your body.
- Lift your hips and bring your knees up to your chest. Bend your elbows and place your hands on each side of your spine to support your lower back.
- As you breathe out, raise your legs and hips to make an angle of roughly 60°. Breathe out, hold your breath and engage your perineum.
- As you breathe in, relax it. Repeat 4 times.
- As you breathe out, bend your knees and bring your thighs towards your stomach.
- Slide your hands towards your buttocks while you gently move your back, bottom and feet to the ground.

Butterfly wings

- Sit cross-legged, lift your head and flutter your eyelids as fast as you can for 30 seconds.
- Close your eyes and lower your head.
- Rub the palms of your hands to create heat.
- Cup your hands over your eyes. Hold them for 5 to 10 breaths. Relax.

Mudra for loving yourself

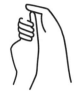

- Point your left index finger. Place your right thumb on your left index finder, then wrap the other fingers from your right hand around it.
- Close your eyes and hold the mudra in front of your chest and breathe deeply for 1 minute. Imagine your left index finger is a fragile, beautiful you. Welcome the feelings.

Visualisation

- Relax your hands on your knees.
- Imagine those close to you taking you in their arms, smiling at you and talking to you with kind, encouraging words. If you want, take your baby in your arms so they can share in the sensations.

Savasana

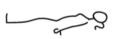

- Lie on your back for the final relaxation, with your legs stretched out in front of you and your arms beside your body with your palms facing upwards.
- Rest for 5 to 10 minutes.

Today's society pushes women to pick up their lives, their rhythm, their pattern, very quickly after childbirth. This return doesn't have to be so quick and brutal, and you have nine months to prepare. Rest as much as you can, take breaks, try not to do any heavy lifting and get help with daily tasks.

Essential oils are not recommended while you are breastfeeding.

Wear some jewellery containing green aventurine or carry some in your pocket to combat the feeling of loss.

Perimenopause and menopause

The menopause is a natural phenomenon which involves the end of periods. It is preceded by the perimenopause, a phase of irregular periods. The menopause is not a disease, even if it often comes with unpleasant symptoms. In Chinese traditional medicine, it is considered a 'second spring'.

If you are troubled by hot flushes, irritability, night sweats and other inconveniences, these postures will help you get over them, while remaining beautiful and fulfilled.

Note down the symptoms you encounter and rate them on a scale of 0 to 10 (0 being the lightest and 10 the most uncomfortable). Follow this session two or three (or more) times per week and compare them every week to see the difference.

....

....

....

....

Sankalpa

- Sit down with your legs crossed.
- Put your palms together and your fingers upright together in front of your chest. Close your eyes.
- Take some deep breaths and speak your intention in a loud voice: 'I am happy to be a beautiful woman.'

Crescent moon

- Get on all fours and place your right foot inside your right hand.
- Anchor to the floor by bending your right knee, making sure it does not go past your ankle.
- As you breathe out, lift your perineum.
- As you breathe in, stretch your arms to the ceiling and feel your chest open up.
- Keep your shoulders down.
- Look straight in front of you and open your heart chakra for 5 to 10 breaths.
- Do the same on the other side.

Garland

- Crouch down with your feet flat on the floor.
- Push your knees out and lean your body gently forward.
- Place your palms together in front of your chest.
- Stretch out your back by pushing your elbows against your knees.
- If you are not on your period, take 5 to 10 dynamic breaths: inflate your stomach as you inhale and relax it as you exhale, to the rhythm of a clock.
- Otherwise, breathe deeply while you open your sacral chakra.

Reclining butterfly

- Lie on your back.
- Bend your knees and open them outwards, keeping the soles of your feet together.

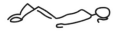

- Place your hands beside your body or on your lower belly in a triangle mudra: only your thumbs and index fingers touch to form a triangle. The other fingers are straight.
- Channel energy to your ovaries and your uterus for 5 to 10 breaths.

Seated twist

- Put your legs out in front of you. Bend your right knee and place your right foot outside your left knee.
- Place your right hand on the floor behind you and your left hand on your right hip.
- As you breathe in, push yourself upwards.
- As you breathe out, turn your right shoulder behind you to look over your right shoulder.
- If you are not on your period, take 5 to 10 dynamic breaths: inflate your stomach as you inhale and relax it as you exhale, to the rhythm of a clock.
- Otherwise, breathe deeply while you open your solar plexus chakra. Do the same on the other side.

Bridge

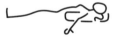

- Lie on your back.
- Bend your knees with your feet hip width apart.
- Keep your arms straight by your body with your palms facing downwards.
- As you breathe out, lift your perineum and push your pelvis upwards. Hold this for 3 to 4 seconds and release as you breathe in.
- Repeat 5 times.

Open heart

- Sit down and place a bolster or a rolled-up blanket behind your back.
- Lie down slowly on the bolster. If you feel tension in your neck, put a cushion under your head.
- Relax your arms and legs.
- Open your heart chakra for 5 to 10 breaths.

Stickers

- Sit cross-legged.
- Raise your eyebrows – without wrinkling your brow – and close your eyes.
- Push your upper eyelids against your lower eyelids for 10 seconds and then release the pressure.
- Repeat twice.

Beautiful skin mudra

· Bend your little fingers and gently press on the nails with your thumbs. The other fingers should point straight upwards.

· Close your eyes and hold your hands at shoulder height while you breathe deeply for 1 minute. Imagine your skin becoming smoother and softer.

Visualisation

· Place your hands gently on your knees.

· Imagine the things you want to do, one by one; people you want to meet, things you want to experience. Go as far as you like with your imagination; a new spring is beginning and anything is possible. Welcome the feelings.

Savasana

· Lie on your back for the final relaxation, with your legs stretched out in front of you and your arms beside your body with your palms facing upwards.

· Rest for 5 to 10 minutes.

Revise your eating habits in order to adapt to your body's changes. Add 'hormone-like' foods to your diet: wheatgerm, wholegrain cereals, cumin, aniseed, sage. Reduce or avoid dairy products, alcohol and sugar completely.

 Inhale or smear between your knuckles a few drops of cypress essential oil to help relieve hot flushes.

Place an orange moonstone on your lower abdomen in the evening and carry it in your pocket during the day to balance your hormonal system.

Overactive thyroid

Hyperthyroidism is linked to the overproduction of hormones by the thyroid gland, situated at the base of the neck. This endocrine gland, shaped like a butterfly, regulates the metabolism of cells and affects weight, mood and the state of your hair and nails. People who suffer from hyperthyroidism are often stressed and hyperactive.

This is reflected in their appearance, movement and even in their attitude. It is therefore essential for them to clear their diaries, to rest and do gentle postures.

This healing will help to calm the throat chakra, which is directly connected to the thyroid gland.

Proceed gently and remember to breathe deeply.

🪷 *Try this session two or three times per week and take note of the physical and emotional changes you experience.*

....

....

....

....

Sankalpa

· Sit down with your legs crossed.
· Put your palms together and your fingers upright together in front of your chest. Close your eyes.
· Take some deep breaths and speak your intention in a loud voice: 'I can listen to to my deepest truths.'

Curled leaf

· Sit on your bended knees.
· Sit back on your heels and keep the tips of your toes together.
· Lower your forehead to the floor, stretch out your back and arms.
· Open your throat chakra for 5 to 10 breaths.

Cow and cat

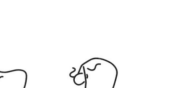

· Get on all fours with your knees hip width apart. Your feet should be relaxed and your hands should be below your shoulders.
· As you breathe in, bend your back down and look up.
· As you breathe out, arch your back and look between your knees.
· Repeat this movement 5 to 10 times and concentrate on the feelings in your throat.

Salamander

· Lie on your front with your hands under your face.
· Relax your hips, legs and feet.
· Take 5 to 10 liberating breaths: breathe in through the nose and out through the mouth, making an 'aaah' sound.

Half-butterfly

· Sit down.
· Put your left leg out in front of you, bend your right knee and open it out. Your right foot should touch the inside of your left thigh.
· Curl your back over forwards and relax your head and arms.
· Open your throat chakra for 5 to 10 breaths. Do the same on the other side.

Sleeping swan

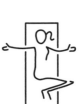

- Straighten your back.
- Bend your left knee and stretch your right leg behind you.
- Place your hands on the floor in front of you. Your left heel should be under your right hip and your left knee should face your right hand.
- Lean gently forwards and put your forehead on the floor, or place a cushion under your forehead. Relax your arms either side of you.
- Take 5 to 10 liberating breaths: breathe in through the nose and out through the mouth, making an 'aaah' sound.
- Repeat on the other side.

Supine twist

- Lie down on your back with your arms out beside you as a cross.
- Bend your knees towards your chest.
- As you breathe out, move your knees to the left as you turn your head to the right. If you feel tension in your lower back, try placing a cushion under your left leg.
- Breathe deeply for 1 minute as you concentrate on your right side. Welcome the relaxing feeling.
- Do the same on the other side.

Rest

- Lie down, feet wide apart on the floor with your knees bent and together.
- Place one hand on your lower abdomen and the other on your chest in order to reconnect with your feelings.
- Breathe deeply 5 to 10 times.

Neck massage

- Sit cross-legged.
- Lift your head gently and slide the tips of your fingers from your chin down to the base of your neck.
- Massage in this way for 1 minute. Imagine you are getting rid of spent energy that has accumulated around your thyroid.

Apana mudra

- Bend your elbows so your hands are at shoulder height.
- Touch the tips of your middle and ring fingers to your thumbs. The other fingers stay straight, pointing upwards.
- Close your eyes and breathe deeply for 1 minute. Imagine you are expelling spent energy like smoke that becomes more and more clear with each breath.

Visualisation

- Put your hands on your knees.
- Concentrate on your throat. Imagine a beautiful sky-blue butterfly. Feed it by breathing for 1 minute and imagine the colour becoming more and more clear with each breath.

Savasana

- Lie on your back for the final relaxation, with your legs stretched out in front of you and your arms beside your body with your palms facing upwards.
- Rest for 5 to 10 minutes.

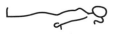

In order to balance your throat chakra and calm your thyroid gland, draw or colour how your spirit feels. Use as many colours as you can. Shut off your inner critic and let yourself go.

- In order to calm your thyroid gland, massage your neck with a mixture of 5 drops of myrrh essential oil and 1 teaspoon of vegetable oil. Massage like this twice a day, five days out of seven, for a few months.

- Wear a black moonstone pendant or place it over your liver to clean out the anger from your system that has accumulated in your throat.

Underactive thyroid

Hypothyroidism is an insufficient production of hormones by the thyroid gland. If you suffer from hypothyroidism you will probably be lacking in energy. Physically, this usually shows as weight gain/excess, brittle hair and nails.

The masculine postures that channel your root chakra and solar plexus chakra will boost your energy. The postures that stimulate your throat chakra will renew the activity in your endocrine gland and fill you with lightness.

Follow this sequence two or three times a week, noting the physical and emotional differences you experience.

....

....

....

Sankalpa

· Sit down with your legs crossed.
· Put your palms together and your fingers upright together in front of your chest. Close your eyes.
· Take some deep breaths and speak your intention in a loud voice: 'I have the strength and determination to speak my own truth.'

Warrior 1

· Stand up with your hands on your hips.
· Take a big step backwards with your left leg and turn it outwards.
· Slowly, try to put your left heel on the floor
· Turn your left hip to the front to keep your hips balanced.
· Bend your right knee but don't let it go further than your ankle.
· Breathe in and stretch your arms up.
· Keep your shoulders down.

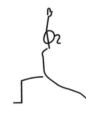

- Keep looking straight in front of you and open your root chakra.
- Do the same on the other side.

Warrior 2

- Keep your left knee bent.
- Turn out your right foot to make a right angle with your left foot.
- Lift your arms so they are parallel with the floor.
- Tense your right leg and look along your left arm.
- Open your solar plexus chakra for 5 to 10 breaths.
- Do the same on the other side.

Tree

- Put your palms together in front of your chest and put your weight on your right foot.
- As you breathe out, lift your perineum and tense your abdominal wall.
- Place your left foot against your right calf or thigh.
- Open your root chakra for 5 to 10 breaths.
- Do the same on the other side.

Dolphin

- Get on all fours.
- Put your forearms on the floor, keeping your elbows below your shoulders and your palms flat on the floor.
- As you breathe out, push the floor with your hands and your forearms.
- Straighten your legs as much as you feel comfortable.
- Take 5 to 10 breaths while you think about the sensations in your throat.

Half-candle

- Lie on your back.
- Bend your knees and place your arms beside your body.
- Lift your hips and bring your knees up to your chest.
- Bend your elbows and place your hands on each side of your spine to support your lower back.
- As you breathe out, raise your legs to make an angle of roughly 60°. Your bodyweight should rest on your shoulders and arms.
- Open your throat chakra for 5 to 10 breaths.

Plough

- Supporting your back with your hands, bend your knees and bring them up towards your face.
- If you can, stretch your legs and place your toes on the floor behind your head.
- Open your throat chakra for 5 to 10 breaths.
- As you breathe out, keeping your knees bent, slide your hands towards your buttocks while gently lowering your back, bottom and feet to the floor.

Fish

- Place your arms beside your body and your hands under your buttocks.
- Breathe in and push your ribcage upwards, maintaining pressure on your buttocks and your forearms.
- Bring your shoulder blades together to arch your back.
- Put the top of your head on the floor without putting pressure on your neck.
- Open your throat chakra for 5 to 10 breaths.
- Slide your head back to place your neck, then your back, on the ground.

Neck loosening

- Sit cross-legged.
- As you breathe in, turn your head gently to the left.
- As you breathe out, turn it to the right. Repeat this movement 3 times.
- As you breathe in, lift your head up gently and as you breathe out, bring your chin down to your chest.
- Repeat this movement 3 times.

Prana mudra

- Bend your elbows to bring your hands to shoulder level.
- Place the tip of your thumb on the tip of your ring finger and little finger. The other fingers stay straight, pointing upwards.
- Breathe deeply for 1 minute. Imagine a light coming down from the sky, entering your body through your forefinger and index finger, and filling your entire body.

Visualisation

- Relax your hands and place them on your knees.
- Concentrate on your throat and imagine a beautiful sky-blue butterfly has landed on it. Feed it with your breath for 1 minute. Imagine the colour becoming more vivid and shiny with each breath.

Savasana

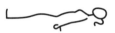

- Lie on your back for the final relaxation, with your legs stretched out in front of you and your arms beside your body with your palms facing upwards.
- Rest for 5 to 10 minutes.

To activate your throat chakra and stimulate your thyroid gland, sing every day. Whisper, hum, shout. Express yourself with your voice.

In order to activate your thyroid gland, massage your neck with a mixture of 5 drops of green myrtle essential oil and 1 teaspoon of vegetable oil. Massage like this twice a day, five days out of seven, for a few months.

Wear a blue chalcedony pendant or hold a crystal in your hands during meditation in order to squeeze out the unspoken things that have accumulated in your throat.

Relationships

Relationships are essential parts of life. They allow us to grow up, understand, communicate and evolve. Each relationship needs to be cultivated and fed, whether it is an emotional relationship, professional relationship, or one with your own self. Love and compassion are the best allies of relationships.

To be comfortable within yourself, learn to listen to your needs, to connect with yourself and to listen to your inner voice.

The sessions in this theme are based around postures that activate your heart chakra and encourage the flow of energy. Be welcoming and let your emotions run free, tears of joy as well as laughter.

Me, my best friend

Your relationship with yourself is at the core of all your relationships. Relationships you develop with others – men or women – are a mirror into how you live within yourself. If you treat yourself with love and respect, you will encounter the same in others. Being good to yourself is the best present you can possibly give.

For some of us, becoming our own best friend is a real challenge. The postures in this session will help you to open up to and love yourself.

Write down two or three ideas for how to express your love for yourself.

....

....

....

....

....

Sankalpa

· Sit down with your legs crossed.
· Put your palms together and your fingers upright together in front of your chest. Close your eyes.
· Take some deep breaths and speak your intention in a loud voice: 'I am my best friend and I am overjoyed about it.'

Salamander

- Lie on your front with your hands under your face. Relax your hips, legs and feet.
- Open your sacral chakra for 5 to 10 breaths.

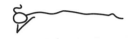

Cobra

- Stretch out your legs and feet.
- Put your hands either side of your ribcage.
- Flatten your feet and lift your perineum.
- As you breathe in, push down with your hands and lift your head, shoulders and chest. Keep your elbows slightly bent and do not lift your shoulders.
- Look in front of you and open your heart chakra for 5 to 10 breaths.
- Put your head back down.

Cat stretch

- Get on all fours. Keep your knees hip width apart and feet flat.
- Walk your hands forward to put your forehead on the floor.
- Open your heart chakra for 5 to 10 breaths.

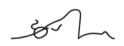

Camel

- Come back upright, keeping your knees on the floor.
- Flatten your feet and place your hands at the base of your back, pointing your fingers upwards.
- As you breathe in, stretch your back.
- As you breathe out, engage your perineum and tilt your pelvis forward, keeping your head upright and tensing your abs.
- If you can, place one hand on one heel then the other on the other heel and tilt your head gently backwards.
- Open your heart chakra for 5 or 10 breaths.
- Come back to position gently.

Downward-facing dog

· Get on all fours, and hook your toes to the floor.
· As you breathe out, push the floor with your hands and toes and lift your pelvis to the ceiling. Keep your knees slightly bent in order to keep your back straight.
· Relax your head, look back between your legs.
· Open your root chakra for 5 to 10 breaths.

Supine twist

· Lie down on your back.
· Place your arms out beside you as a cross.
· Bend your knees towards your chest.
· As you breathe out, move your knees to the left as you turn your head to the right. If you feel tension in your lower back, try placing a cushion under your left leg.
· Breathe deeply for 1 minute, concentrating on your right side. Relax.
· Do the same on the other side.

Hug

· Bend your knees with your feet on the floor, at least hip width apart, knees touching.
· Cross your arms over your chest to hold yourself in your arms.
· Stay in this position for 1 minute while breathing deeply.
· Whisper gentle words of well-being to yourself.

Sky kisses

· Sit cross-legged.
· Tilt your head gently backwards, taking care of your neck.
· Kiss upwards with an exaggerated movement.
· Repeat 9 times.

Heart connection mudra

· Place your left hand in the centre of your chest, then the right hand over it.

· Close your eyes and breathe deeply for 1 minute. Listen to your heart and accept the woman that you are with all your strengths and weaknesses.

Visualisation

· Place your hands on your knees.

· Think about a situation where you looked after yourself as you would have a friend. Let these happy feelings take hold.

Savasana

· Lie on your back for the final relaxation, with your legs stretched out in front of you and your arms beside your body with your palms facing upwards.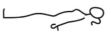

· Rest for 5 to 10 minutes.

Being familiar with your needs helps you better understand who you are and where your limits lie. Make a list of your physical, material and emotional needs. Think about how you can satisfy them and communicate them to others.

In order to intensify your feeling of inner peace, spray frankincense oil around you.

Wear some lemon chrysoprase jewellery, carry the crystal in your pocket or hold it in your hands during meditation in order to reinforce your love for yourself.

Contact with others

Interaction with other people contributes to our emotional, intellectual and professional development. If you are usually solitary or naturally prefer to be alone, take care not to isolate yourself or shut yourself away.

The postures that stimulate the heart chakra will help you open up to others. The postures for the throat chakra will help you to better express your needs.

🪷 *Note down how you are when you meet a new person. How could you do better?*

....

....

....

....

Sankalpa

· Sit down with your legs crossed.
· Put your palms together and your fingers upright together in front of your chest. Close your eyes.
· Take some deep breaths and speak your intention in a loud voice: 'I open my heart to new things and I accept them with pleasure.'

Tiger

· Get on all fours with your knees hip width apart. Your feet should be flat and your hands should be below your shoulders.
· As you breathe in, lift your left leg up and bend your back gently.
· As you breathe out, bring the knee to the front while arching your back.
· Repeat 4 times on each side while opening your sacral chakra.

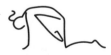

Crescent moon

- Place your right foot inside your right hand.
- Anchor to the floor by bending your right knee, making sure it does not go past your ankle.
- As you breathe out, lift your perineum.
- As you breathe in, stretch your arms to the ceiling with your palms touching.
- Keep your shoulders down.
- Look straight in front of you and feed your heart chakra for 5 to 10 breaths.
- Do the same on the other side.

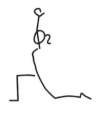

Cosmic dancer

- Stand up and put your bodyweight on your left foot.
- Bend your left knee.
- Put your left foot in your left hand and lift it behind you.
- Hold out your right arm horizontally, look down your right arm and bend gently forwards to maintain balance.
- Open your heart chakra for 5 to 10 breaths.
- Do the same on the other side.

Caterpillar

- Sit down with your legs out straight in front of you.
- As you breathe out, bring your upper body forwards to your legs. Keep your legs and arms relaxed.
- Open your throat chakra for 5 to 10 breaths.

Half-candle

- Lie on your back.
- Bend your knees and lie your arms beside your body.
- Lift your hips and bring your knees up to your chest.
- Bend your elbows and place your hands on each side of your spine to support your lower back.
- As you breathe out, raise your legs and hips to make an angle of roughly 60°. Your bodyweight should now be on your shoulders and arms.
- Open your throat chakra for 5 to 10 breaths.

Plough

- Supporting your back with your hands, bend your knees and bring them up towards your face.
- If you can, stretch your legs and place your toes on the floor behind your head.
- Open your throat chakra for 5 to 10 breaths.
- As you breathe out, keeping your knees bent, slide your hands towards your buttocks while gently lowering your back, bottom and feet to the floor.

Open heart

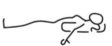

- Sit down and place a bolster or a rolled-up blanket behind your back.
- Lie down slowly on the bolster. If you feel tension in your neck, put a cushion under your head. Relax your arms and legs.
- Open your heart chakra for 5 to 10 breaths.

Lion breathing

- Sit cross-legged. Breathe in deeply, close your eyes and hold your fists in front of your chest.
- Breathe out powerfully from your mouth. At the same time, stick out your tongue, open your eyes and look up between your eyebrows, opening your fists and stretching out your fingers.
- Repeat 2 times.

Shell mudra

- Wrap your left thumb in the fingers of your right hand.
- Place your right thumb on the straightened middle finger of your left hand.
- Close your eyes and hold the mudra at throat level. Breathe deeply for 1 minute. Imagine a blue light coming from your throat and channelling through the shell to the outside world. Welcome the feelings.

Visualisation

- Place your hands on your knees. Think about one or two people you would like to know.
- Imagine you are talking to them happily. Take note of the feelings.

Savasana

- Lie on your back for the final relaxation, with your legs stretched out in front of you and your arms beside your body with your palms facing upwards.

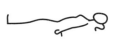

- Rest for 5 to 10 minutes.

Our thoughts influence ourselves but also those around us. Smile and be polite and friendly to people you meet, greeting them warmly and wishing them well. You will notice a difference on the inside and the outside.

Massage your solar plexus with a mixture of 1 drop of bergamot essential oil and 4 drops of vegetable oil to strengthen your self-confidence.

Wear a blue topaz pendant to strengthen your social relationships and enable you to mix freely with others.

Professional relationships

Relationships at work can be truly challenging, especially if the person that induces stress is your superior or your subordinate. Although working in a team is not always easy, because we can't always have things our way, it is much more fulfilling to work together than on your own. As the saying goes: if you want to go fast, go alone; if you want to go far, go together.

The postures in this sequence will help you stay true to your nature, be convincing when needed, and concentrate on creating harmonious relationships in your workplace.

✿ Write down the names of a co-worker with whom you would like to improve your relationship. How can you do this?

....

....

....

....

....

Sankalpa

· Sit down with your legs crossed.
· Put your palms together and your fingers upright together in front of your chest. Close your eyes.
· Take some deep breaths and speak your intention in a loud voice: 'I am filled with gratitude for the harmonious relationships with my co-workers.'

Triangle

- Take a big step back with your right foot and turn it out to make a right angle with your left foot.
- Straighten your arms at shoulder height, keeping them parallel to the floor.
- As you breathe out, lift your perineum and keep your hips forward.
- Bend over to the left and put your left hand on your shin.
- Stretch your right hand to the ceiling.
- Open your root chakra for 5 to 10 breaths.
- Do the same on the other side.

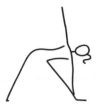

Tree

- Put your palms together in front of your chest and put your weight on your right foot.
- As you breathe out, lift your perineum and tense your abdominal wall.
- Place your left foot against your right calf.
- Open your root chakra for 5 to 10 breaths then do the same on the other side.

Boat

- Sit down.
- Bend your knees and hold the backs of your thighs with your hands.
- Tense your perineum and your abdominal wall.
- As you breathe out, raise your feet one by one to have your shins parallel with the floor. If this is easy, release your hands and hold your arms out so they are parallel to the floor.
- Open your solar plexus chakra for 5 to 10 breaths.

Seated twist

- Put your left leg out in front. Bend your right knee and place your right foot outside your left knee.
- Place your right hand on the floor behind you and your left hand on your right hip.
- As you breathe in, push yourself upwards and, as you breathe out, turn your right shoulder behind you.

- Look over your right shoulder.
- If you are not on your period, take 5 to 10 dynamic breaths: inflate your stomach as you inhale and relax it as you exhale, to the rhythm of a clock.
- Otherwise, breathe deeply and open your solar plexus chakra, then change knees and repeat on the other side.

Half-candle

- Lie on your back.
- Bend your knees and place your arms beside your body.
- Lift your hips and bring your knees up to your chest.
- Bend your elbows and place your hands on each side of your spine to support your lower back.
- As you breathe out, raise your legs to make an angle of roughly 60°.
- Your bodyweight should rest on your shoulders and arms.
- Open your throat chakra for 5 to 10 breaths.

Locust

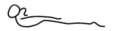

- Lie on your chest, keep your legs together and keep your front on the floor.
- Link your fingers behind your back.
- Bring your shoulder blades together, keeping your arms straight.
- As you breathe out, lift your perineum.
- Lift your head and chest, keeping your instep on the floor and pushing your hands in the direction of your feet.
- Feed your heart chakra for 5 to 10 breaths.

Rain on the face

- Sit in a comfortable position.
- Close your eyes for 1 minute then tap lightly with the tips of your fingers starting from the base of the neck, moving gradually upwards to the forehead and then going back to the base of the neck. Repeat a few times.

Poise mudra

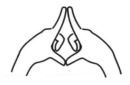

- Bend your middle fingers, ring fingers and little fingers.
- Stretch your index fingers and thumbs out as much as you can and touch the tips together.
- Close your eyes and hold the mudra in front of your solar plexus. Your thumbs should point towards the body.
- Breathe deeply for 1 minute and feel the confidence building inside you.

Visualisation

- Release the mudra and put your hands on your knees.
- Visualise your day at work, going through each detail starting from the morning when you enter your workplace and finishing with the moment you leave for home. Every time you see the co-worker with whom you would like to improve your relationship, imagine that you give them a flower or another pretty object, and they accept it with joy and gratitude.
- Feel free to repeat this joyful visualisation during the day at work and observe the positive changes in your co-worker's behavior.

Savasana

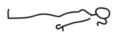

- Lie on your back for the final relaxation, with your legs stretched out in front of you and your arms beside your body with your palms facing upwards.
- Rest for 5 to 10 minutes.

You never know what another person is going through, so don't jump to conclusions when your co-worker acts unpleasantly. Ask instead if everything is okay, and if they need help. Given that good deeds have a tendency to be reciprocal, you might be the one who will benefit from this next time.

- Apply 1 drop of silver-fir essential oil on the inner side of each wrist and inhale it deeply to prevent burn-out, and gain courage and willpower.

- To reinforce your personal space and be able to say, 'No' when needed, wear a bronzite crystal in your pocket or as jewellery.

A fulfilling relationship

Love, forgiveness and communication are the main ingredients for a stable, fulfilling relationship. Grudges that we build up throughout our lives can prevent us from having a truly loving experience.

This session contains postures for your heart chakra, in order to relieve your feelings. The postures for your sacral chakra will light the flames of passion.

Stay in touch with your feelings and your emotions.

🪷 *Take note of your feelings and emotions before and after the session.*

....

....

....

....

Sankalpa

· Sit down with your legs crossed.
· Put your palms together and your fingers upright together in front of your chest. Close your eyes.
· Take some deep breaths and speak your intention in a loud voice: 'I let love and passion flow all around my loving relationship.'

Goddess

· As you breathe in, open your arms wide and look up.
· As you breathe out, lower your head and wrap yourself in your arms. Repeat 5 or 6 times.

Stretch twist

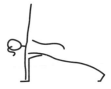

· Get on all fours.
· Put your right foot inside your right hand.
· Turn out the toes on your left foot to aid stability.
· Put your left hand on the floor inside your left foot.
· Raise your right hand upwards.
· Stretch both hands as you push against the floor. If you are comfortable, tense your left leg.
· Look in front of you, upwards.
· If it is not your period, take 5 to 10 dynamic breaths: inflate your stomach as you inhale and relax it as you exhale, to the rhythm of a clock.
· Otherwise breathe deeply, channelling your sacral chakra and do the same on the other side.

Cat stretch

· Put your knees on the floor, hip-width apart.
· Relax your feet.
· Walk your hands forward to put your forehead on the floor.
· Open your heart chakra for 5 to 10 breaths.

Pelvic rotation

· Stand up with your feet hip width apart.
· Put your hands on your hips.
· Rotate your hips in circles.
· Do the movement 10 times one way then 10 times the other.

Ragdoll

· Place your feet hip width apart, knees bent.
· As you breathe out, completely relax your upper body.
· Bend your elbows and hold them in your hands.
· If it is not your period, take 5 to 10 dynamic breaths: inflate your stomach as you inhale and relax it as you exhale, to the rhythm of a clock.
· Otherwise breathe deeply, channelling your sacral chakra.

Cobra

· Lie on your front.
· Keep your feet and legs together and put your hands either side of your ribcage.
· Flatten your feet and lift your perineum.
· As you breathe in, push down with your hands and lift your head, shoulders and chest. Keep your elbows bent and do not lift your shoulders.
· Look in front of you and open your heart chakra for 5 to 10 breaths.
· Put your head back down.

Reclining butterfly with support

· Sit down and place a bolster or rolled-up blanket at the base of your spine.
· Lie slowly back onto the bolster. If you feel tension in the neck, put a cushion under your head.

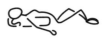

· Bend your knees and open them outwards, keeping the soles of your feet together.
· Breathe deeply. Imagine that air is entering and exiting from the centre of your chest for 5 to 10 breaths.

Natural blusher

· Sit cross-legged.
· Pinch your cheeks lightly with your fingertips and thumb. Start at your cheekbones and go down as far as your lower jaw.
· Repeat 3 times.

Mudra of union

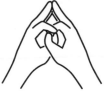

- Join the tips of your index finger and thumb of your right hand and put them inside the same circle of your left hand so it looks like two linked rings. The tips of your other fingers should be touching and pointing upwards.
- Close your eyes and hold the mudra at chest level while you breathe deeply for 1 minute. Imagine the person you love is in front of you. Feel the love and passion flowing around you.

Visualisation

- Relax your hands on your knees or thighs.
- Imagine a ray of pink light linking your heart with the person you love. This light represents the love you feel for each other. Let your partner's light fill you completely; welcome it.

Savasana

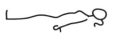

- Lie on your back for the final relaxation, with your legs stretched out in front of you and your arms beside your body with your palms facing upwards.
- Rest for 5 to 10 minutes.

Each relationship needs new things in order to be fulfilled. Make time for yourselves as a couple, one evening per week for example. Make the most of it to go out together, go for a walk, find a new restaurant. If you are single, spend this time with a friend.

Spray ylang-ylang essential oil around you to better express your emotions and your sensuality.

Wear some jewellery with blue sapphire in it, or carry the stone in your pocket to attract your partner.

Reconnect with your inner child

The inner child is a part of us that holds on to joy, creativity and spontaneity. It is light, carefree and allows us to overcome obstacles with optimism.

This session allows you to understand the stages of a child's physical and emotional development in order to reconnect with it. Starting with the development as a foetus in the mother's uterus, it then grows and lays down its own roots in the outside world.

Be aware or your feelings during this internal journey.

Note down the words or feelings of your inner child after the session.

....

....

....

....

Sankalpa

· Sit down with your legs crossed.
· Put your palms together and your fingers upright together in front of your chest. Close your eyes.
· Take some deep breaths and speak your intention in a loud voice: 'I devote time to my inner child and I nourish them with love.'

Foetus

- Bend your knees and roll over to your right side.
- Put your arms under your head.
- Feed your heart chakra for 5 to 10 breaths.

Child

- Sit on your heels with your knees and feet bent.
- Lower your forehead to the floor, keeping your arms by your sides.
- Feed your heart chakra for 5 to 10 breaths.

Locust

- Lie on your chest.
- Keep your legs together and keep your front on the floor.
- Link your fingers behind your back and bring your shoulder blades together, keeping your arms straight.
- As you breathe out, lift your perineum.
- Lift your head and chest, keeping your instep on the floor and pushing your hands in the direction of your feet.
- Feed your heart chakra for 5 to 10 breaths.

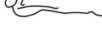

Cow and cat

- Get on all fours. Your knees should not be wider than your hips. Your feet should be flat and your hands should be below your shoulders.
- As you breathe in, bend your back down and look up.
- As you breathe out, arch your back and look between your knees.
- Repeat this movement 5 to 10 times as you open your heart chakra.

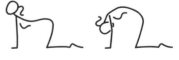

Downward-facing dog

- Hook your toes to the floor.
- As you breathe out, push the floor with your hands and toes.
- Lift your pelvis towards the ceiling. Keep your knees slightly bent in order to keep your back straight.
- Relax your head, look back between your legs.
- Open your root chakra for 5 to 10 breaths.

Ragdoll

- Walk towards your hands and place your feet hip width apart.
- Bend your knees and completely relax your upper body.
- Bend your elbows and hold them in your hands.
- Take 5 to 10 deep breaths.

Tree

- Roll your back up slowly and stand up. Put your palms together in front of your chest.
- Put your weight on your right foot.
- As you breathe out, lift your perineum and tense your abdominal wall.
- Place your left foot against your right calf.
- Open your root chakra for 5 to 10 breaths.
- Do the same on the other side.

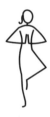

Eyebrow massage

- Sit down with your legs crossed and bend your index fingers.
- Slide your knuckles across your eyebrows, from inside to out.
- Repeat the massage 9 times.

Contemplation mudra

· Put your right hand in your left hand with your palms facing upwards. Your hands should be relaxed and thumbs should be touching.

· Close your eyes and hold the mudra in front of your lower body as you breathe deeply for 1 minute. Imagine you are cradling your inner child. Welcome the feelings.

Visualisation

· Relax your hands on your knees or thighs.

· Imagine yourself as a child. Look at the expression on your face. Approach the child and take them in your arms. Tell them you love them and that you will always be there for them. Take notice of any changes this provokes.

Savasana

· Lie on your back for the final relaxation, with your legs stretched out in front of you and your arms beside your body with your palms facing upwards.

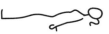

· Rest for 5 to 10 minutes.

---

*Like all children, the inner child likes to have fun.
Bring more joy and creativity into your life.
Use coloured pencils in your diary, sing, dance, play.*

Massage your solar plexus, your inner wrists and the arches of your feet with 3 to 4 drops of mandarin essential oil in order to reconnect with your inner child.

Each evening, place a morganite on your stomach to heal your inner child.

Relationships with children

What could be more fun than a yoga session with your children? Invite them on to the mat and tell them this story, accompanied by the postures in this session.

A peaceful warrior is hunting for treasure. He gets ready to leave one night and departs at dawn. On the horizon he sees a big tree and approaches it. Behind the tree is a calm lake with a bridge across it. The warrior crosses the bridge and gets into the boat berthed next to it.

A swan glides past on the water just beside him. A little fish swims past peacefully and leaps in the water. The sun rises gently in the distance. Insects come out to sing their morning song. A glinting blue dragonfly flies over the lake. A bee buzzes as it collects nectar from the flowers. After many hours, the warrior finally encounters the treasure: a beautiful lotus floating on the water.

After the session, note down the postures that your children liked.

....

....

....

Sankalpa

· Sit down with your legs crossed.
· Put your palms together and your fingers upright together in front of your chest. Close your eyes.
· Take some deep breaths and speak your intention in a loud voice: 'I am a peaceful warrior who brings light to the lives of others.'

Warrior 2

- Stand upright.
- Take a big step back with your left foot and turn it out to make a right angle with the right foot.
- Lift your arms so they are parallel with the floor.
- Bend your right knee but do not let it go past your shin.
- Engage your right leg and look along your left arm.
- Open your root chakra for 5 to 10 breaths.
- Do the same on the other side.

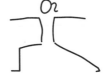

Tree

- Stand up and put your palms together in front of your chest.
- Put your weight on your right foot.
- As you breathe out, lift your perineum and tense your abdominal wall.
- Place your left foot against your right calf.
- Open your root chakra for 5 to 10 breaths.
- Do the same on the other side.

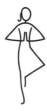

Bridge

- Lie on your back, bend your knees with your feet hip width apart.
- Keep your arms straight by your body with your palms facing downwards.
- Breathe out, lift your perineum and push your pelvis upwards.
- Open your root chakra for 5 to 10 breaths.

Boat

- Sit down, bend your knees and hold the backs of your thighs with your hands.
- Tense your perineum and your abdominal wall.
- As you breathe out, raise your feet one by one until your shins are parallel with the floor.
- If you are comfortable, release your hands and hold your arms out.
- Open your solar plexus chakra for 5 to 10 breaths.

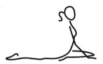

Swan

- Place your left knee on the floor and place your left foot in front of your right hip.
- Stretch your right leg out behind you, keeping your instep flat on the floor.
- Place your hands each side of your hips and open your chest. If you tilt to the left, place a cushion under your left buttock.
- Open your heart chakra for 5 to 10 breaths.

Fish

- Lie on your back and place your arms beside your body and your hands under your buttocks.
- Breathe in and push your ribcage upwards, maintaining pressure on your buttocks and your forearms.
- Bring your shoulder blades together to arch your back.
- Put the top of your head on the floor without putting pressure on your neck.
- Open your throat chakra for 5 to 10 breaths.
- Slide your head back to place your neck, then your back, on the ground.

Dragonfly

- Sit down with your legs apart in front of you.
- Place a cushion in front of you to go beneath your upper body.
- As you breathe out, lean gently forward. Your back should be relaxed and curved.
- Open your sacral chakra for 5 to 10 breaths.

Bee breathing

- Sit cross-legged.
- Plug your ears with your index fingers and close your eyes.
- Breathe in deeply and exhale as you make a 'mmm' sound.
- Repeat 3 times.

Lotus mudra

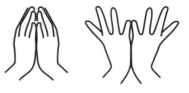

- Put your hands together in front of your solar plexus. Only the sides of the hands and the tips of your fingers should be touching, to make a closed lotus.
- Gently lift the lotus towards your heart and then throat. Keep lifting your hands to your face as you open them up. The tips of your little fingers, your thumbs and your wrists should be touching. The lotus leaves the water and opens in the sun. Keep the lotus in front of your forehead and take 5 to 10 deep breaths. Imagine a luminous, shiny lotus that lights up others with its purity.

Savasana

- Lie on your back for the final relaxation, with your legs stretched out in front of you and your arms beside your body with your palms facing upwards.
- Rest for 5 to 10 minutes.

Children are the best teachers. They have a strong, natural link to the cosmos. They know precisely what is good for them and for others. When you are annoyed with your children, think about how you can make things better in order to become a better version of yourself.

Most essential oils are not recommended for children under six. Even so, you could atomise a mist of lavender oil around before the session, for calmness.

To allow all aspects of your children to grow, give a blue moonstone to girls and a sunstone to boys.

Relief from emotional pain

Emotional wounds can be deeply rooted in our spirit and our body. Learn to forgive to have a fulfilled life. If forgiving is difficult, be patient and give yourself time to heal your broken heart.

The postures in this session will help you to let go, and to accept and liberate yourself.

🪷 *On a scale of 0 to 10 (0 being the least and 10 the most painful), measure your emotional pain. Evaluate it again after the session.*

....

....

....

....

....

Sankalpa

- Sit down with your legs crossed.
- Put your palms together and your fingers upright together in front of your chest. Close your eyes.
- Take some deep breaths and speak your intention in a loud voice: 'I recognise the power of my heart, which is ready to forgive.'

Curled leaf

- Sit on your knees and open them out.
- Sit back on your heels and keep the tips of your toes together.
- Lower your forehead to the floor, stretch out your back and arms.
- Open your heart chakra for 5 to 10 breaths.

Open heart

- Get up, sit and place a bolster or a rolled-up blanket behind your back.
- Lie down slowly on the bolster. If you feel tension in your neck, put a cushion under your head.
- Relax your arms and legs.
- Open your heart chakra for 5 to 10 breaths. Let the pain out of your heart.

Foetus

- Bend your knees and roll over to your right side.
- Put your arms under your head.
- Feed your heart chakra for 5 to 10 breaths.

Downward-facing dog

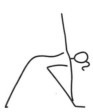

- Get on all fours, and hook your toes to the floor.
- As you breathe out, push the floor with your hands and toes and lift your pelvis to the ceiling. Keep your knees slightly bent in order to keep your back straight.
- Relax your head, look back between your legs.
- Open your root chakra for 5 to 10 breaths.

Triangle

- Stand up straight.
- Take a big step back with your right foot and turn it out to make a right angle with your left foot.
- Straighten your arms to shoulder height, keeping them parallel to the floor.

- As you breathe out, lift your perineum.
- Bend over to the left and put your left hand on your left shin, keeping your hips facing forward.
- Stretch your right hand to the ceiling.
- Open your root chakra for 5 to 10 breaths.
- Do the same on the other side.

Aeroplane

- Stand upright with the weight of your body on your right foot and straighten your arms.
- As you breathe out, lift your perineum and tense your abdominal wall. Lean over frontwards by lifting your left leg until your body and left leg are both parallel with the floor.
- Take 5 to 10 breaths as you keep balanced, then do the same on the other side.

Warrior 1

- Take a big step backwards with your left leg and turn it outwards.
- Slowly, try to put your left heel on the floor.
- Turn your left hip to the front to keep your hips balanced.
- Bend your right knee but don't let it go further than your ankle.
- Breathe in and stretch your arms up.
- Keep your shoulders down.
- Keep looking straight in front of you and open your root chakra.
- Do the same on the other side.

Temple massage

- Sit cross-legged.
- Put the tips of your index and middle fingers on your temples.
- Make 5 to 10 circular movements to the front, then 5 to 10 to the back.

Alternate breathing

· Put your left hand on your knee.
· Touch the space between your eyebrows with the tips of your index and middle fingers of your right hand.
· Seal your right nostril with the thumb and breathe in through your left nostril.
· Seal your left nostril with your little finger, open your right nostril and breathe out through it.
· Alternate your breathing for 2 to 5 cycles.

Visualisation

· Relax your hands on your knees or thighs.
· Imagine someone that you hurt in front of you. Many coloured threads join you to this person. The threads represent the different aspects of your interactions with them. Take a pair of imaginary scissors and cut the threads one by one. When all have been cut, that person may depart in peace. Welcome the new life that awaits you.

Savasana

· Lie on your back for the final relaxation, with your legs stretched out in front of you and your arms beside your body with your palms facing upwards.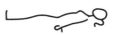
· Rest for 5 to 10 minutes.

Take time to forgive yourself. Write yourself a letter asking for forgiveness for what you have done, or not done. Then write yourself a second letter forgiving yourself.

Massage your solar plexus and the inside of your wrists with a mixture of 1 drop of damask rose essential oil and 10 drops of vegetable oil. The mixture will help you overcome your wounds and find your inner peace.

Wear some jewellery with kunzite in it. Carry some in your pocket or hold some in your hand during meditation to make it easier to forgive.

Accepting solitude

Moments of isolation are necessary to reconnect with yourself, to heal the wounds of the past, to understand your needs and to learn how to better communicate with others.

If a feeling of loneliness persists and becomes difficult, allow yourself some time for introspection.

Loneliness gives us a feeling of emptiness that we want to fill with love. Touch this emptiness and fill it, using the postures for your root chakra (strength), sacral (acceptance) and heart (love).

🪷 *Make a note of the times in which you feel particularly alone. What is that loneliness trying to tell you?*

....

....

....

Sankalpa

· Sit down with your legs crossed.
· Put your palms together and your fingers upright together in front of your chest. Close your eyes.
· Take some deep breaths and speak your intention in a loud voice: 'I welcome time spent with myself.'

Half-butterfly

· Put your left leg out in front of you, bend your right knee and open it out. Your right foot should touch the inside of your left thigh.
· Curl your back over forwards and relax your head and arms.
· Open your root chakra for 5 to 10 breaths.
· Do the same on the other side.

Tiger

- Get on all fours with your knees hip width apart. Your feet should be flat and your hands should be below your shoulders.
- As you breathe in, lift your left leg up and bend your back gently.
- As you breathe out, bring the knee to the front while arching your back. Repeat 4 times on each side as you open your sacral chakra.

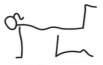
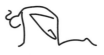

Warrior 2

- Stand up.
- Take a big step back with your left foot and turn it out to make a right angle with the right foot.
- Lift your arms so they are parallel with the floor.
- Bend your right knee but do not let it go past your ankle.
- Engage your left leg and look along the length of your right arm.
- Take 5 to 10 breaths, imagining a light coming out of your heart and your hands.
- Do the same on the other side.

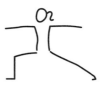

Fish

- Lie on your back.
- Place your arms beside your body and your hands under your buttocks.
- Breathe in and push your ribcage upwards, maintaining pressure on your buttocks and your forearms.
- Bring your shoulder blades together to arch your back.
- Put the top of your head on the floor without putting pressure on your neck.
- Open your heart chakra for 5 to 10 breaths.
- Slide your head back to place your neck, then your back, on the ground.

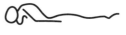

Seed

- Bring your legs to your chest and wrap your arms around them.
- If you are not on your period, take 5 to 10 dynamic breaths: inflate your stomach as you inhale and relax it as you exhale, to the rhythm of a clock.
- Otherwise, breathe deeply and open your sacral chakra.

Camel

- Sit on your knees.
- Place your hands at the base of your back, pointing your fingers upwards.
- As you breathe in, stretch your back.
- As you breathe out, lift your perineum and tilt your pelvis forward, keeping your head upright. Keep your perineum and abs tensed.
- If you can, place one hand on one heel then the other on the other heel and tilt your head gently backwards.
- Open your heart chakra for 5 or 10 breaths and then come back to position gently.

Supported bridge

- Lie on your back.
- Bend your knees and gently lift your hips and slide a cushion or bolster underneath.
- Widen the space between your feet and bring your knees together.
- Open your sacral chakra for 5 to 10 breaths.

Hand on forehead

- Sit cross-legged.
- Tilt your head to one side or tip it forward.
- Place one hand on your forehead, as if someone was touching you and telling you everything was all right.
- Close your eyes and take a few deep breaths as you let the calm settle in.

Mudra of friendship

- Put your hands in front of your chest.
- Place the tips of your thumbs at the base of your ring fingers.
- Roll your ring fingers and middle fingers around them.
- Cross your little fingers and touch the tips of your index fingers, pointing them upwards.
- Close your eyes and hold the mudra in front of your chest while breathing deeply for 1 minute.
- Imagine you are walking down a street and that everybody you pass smiles at you. Welcome the feelings.

Visualisation

- Relax your hands on your knees.
- Concentrate on the middle of your chest and imagine a beautiful green lotus there. Feed it by breathing for 1 minute. Imagine the colour becoming more vivid and intense with each breath.

Savasana

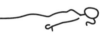

- Lie on your back for the final relaxation, with your legs stretched out in front of you and your arms beside your body with your palms facing upwards.
- Rest for 5 to 10 minutes.

Transform your moments of loneliness into a meeting with yourself. Read books, listen to podcasts, watch personal development videos and learn new things, widen your horizons. Make the most of your own company to evolve and be fulfilled.

Massage your solar plexus, your inner wrists and the arches of your feet with 2 to 3 drops of petitgrain essential oil for a feeling of completeness.

Carry some thulite in your pocket to feel better about yourself and to keep your heart open.

Connecting with nature

Nature influences and transforms women without them even knowing. The biggest factors of these physical and emotional changes are the seasons and the moon.

Women are very sensitive to that astral body. There are eight lunar phases in a 29-day cycle (the same approximate length of a menstrual cycle). For simplicity we list four phases: new moon, crescent moon, full moon and waning moon. These stages play an important role in our physical and psychological health.

These sessions will help you to better connect to yourself during each phase and each season to make the most of the different energies.

New moon

During the new moon phase, the moon is precisely located between the earth and the sun, making it invisible. This only lasts an instant, but it is possible to feel its influence a day before and a day afterwards (tiredness, sleeplessness, anguish, desire to be alone, sadness).

The new moon symbolises renewal and new things. Think about your plans and the projects you want to achieve during the next phase. Sow the seeds now.

The postures in this session activate your sacral chakra and your heart chakra to give you a better connection to solar energy and to better understand your desires.

☙ Make a note of the project you want to work on over the next two weeks.

....

....

....

....

Sankalpa

- Sit down with your legs crossed.
- Put your palms together and your fingers upright together in front of your chest. Close your eyes.
- Take some deep breaths and speak your intention in a loud voice: 'Today I reconnect with my heart and receive an answer to my questions.'

Goddess

- Sit cross-legged, open out your arms as you breathe in and look up to be open to new things.
- As you breathe out, place your hands on your chest to welcome the new project to your heart.

Crescent moon

- Get on all fours.
- Place your right foot inside your right hand. Anchor to the floor by bending your right knee, making sure it does not go past your ankle.
- As you breathe out, lift your perineum.
- As you breathe in, stretch your arms to the ceiling with your palms together.
- Keep your shoulders down.
- Look straight in front of you and open your heart chakra for 5 to 10 breaths.
- Do the same on the other side.

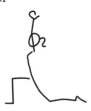

Garland

- Crouch down with your feet flat on the floor. If you cannot do this, place a folded blanket beneath your heels.
- Push your knees out and lean your body gently forward.
- Push out your arms while pushing your elbows against your legs. Put your hands together and put them on the floor
- Relax your head. Imagine you are planting the seed of your next project.
- Hold the position for 5 to 10 breaths.

Cosmic dancer

- Stand up and put your bodyweight on your right foot.
- Bend your left knee.
- Put your left foot in your left hand and lift it behind you.
- Hold out your right arm horizontally, look down your right arm and bend gently forwards to keep balanced.
- Open your heart chakra for 5 to 10 breaths.
- Do the same on the other side.

Locust

- Lie on your chest.
- Keep your legs together and keep your front on the floor.
- Link your fingers behind your back and bring your shoulder blades together, keeping your arms straight.
- As you breathe out, lift your perineum.
- Lift your head and chest, keeping your instep on the floor and pushing your hands in the direction of your feet.
- Feed your heart chakra for 5 to 10 breaths.

Dragonfly

- Sit down with your legs apart in front of you.
- Place a cushion in front of you to go beneath your upper body.
- As you breathe out, lean gently forward. Your back should be relaxed and curved.
- Open your sacral chakra for 5 to 10 breaths.

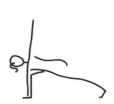

Stretch twist

- Get on all fours.
- Put your right foot inside your right hand.
- Turn out the toes on your left foot to aid stability.
- Put your left hand on the floor inside your left foot and raise your right hand upwards.
- Stretch both hands as you push on the floor. If you are comfortable, tense your left leg.
- Look in front of you, upwards.
- Open your sacral chakra for 5 to 10 breaths.
- Change to the other knee.

Fork

- Sit cross-legged.
- Place your index finger and middle finger of one hand on the bridge of your nose.

- Breathe in deeply.
- As you breathe out, move your fingers up, separate them and push up the skin between your eyebrows.
- Repeat 5 times.

Root lock

- Stay cross-legged and put your hands on your knees or hips.
- As you breathe out, lift your perineum, imagining a spark coming from your coccyx up the length of your spine to your head.
- Repeat 2 to 5 times.

Visualisation

- Imagine now that the spark moves from your coccyx to the top of your head. A fountain of light gushes from your body. For 1 minute, bathe in this light.

Savasana

- Lie on your back for the final relaxation, with your legs stretched out in front of you and your arms beside your body with your palms facing upwards.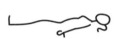
- Rest for 5 to 10 minutes.

During the new moon, our energy is at its lowest. This pausing causes a loss of energy, a worsening of mood and difficulties in communication. Be patient. Do not rush into situations that will cause you to lose energy. Take time for yourself and rest.

Take a hot bath with 10 drops of grapefruit essential oil added to it to revitalise you.

Carry some green aventurine in your pocket, or hold some in your hands during meditation, to help clear your mind and make decisions.

Crescent moon

The crescent moon comprises three phases and lasts 14 days. Over two weeks, more of the moon's surface is gradually revealed until the full moon.

In order to identify a crescent moon, imagine a straight line down the centre. Only the right side will be visible, combining with your finger to make a letter 'p' (as in premier, or first, quarter).

The dominating characteristic of this phase is consistent growing energy. Channel it with this session to sow the seeds of your plans.

🪷 *Note down the stages of achieving your plans.*

....

....

....

....

....

Sankalpa

· Sit down with your legs crossed.
· Put your palms together and your fingers upright together in front of your chest. Close your eyes.
· Take some deep breaths and speak your intention in a loud voice: 'I harness the power of the moon to achieve my plans and I am grateful.'

Cow and cat

- Get on all fours with your knees hip width apart. Your feet should be relaxed and your hands should be below your shoulders.

- As you breathe in, bend your back down and look up.
- As you breathe out, arch your back and look between your knees.
- Repeat this movement 5 to 10 times as you open your heart chakra.

Dolphin

- Put your forearms on the floor, keeping your elbows below your shoulders and your palms flat on the floor.

- As you breathe out, push the floor with your hands and your forearms.
- Straighten your legs as much as you feel comfortable.
- Take 5 to 10 breaths while you think about the sensations in your chest and arms.

Ragdoll

- Walk your feet forward and keep your feet hip width apart.
- Bend your knees and completely relax your upper body.
- Bend your elbows and hold them in your hands.
- Take 5 to 10 deep breaths.

Crescent moon

- Get on all fours.
- Place your right foot inside of your right hand. Anchor to the floor by bending your right knee, making sure it does not go past your ankle.
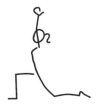
- As you breathe out, lift your perineum.
- As you breathe in, stretch your arms to the ceiling.
- Keep your shoulders down.
- Look straight in front of you and feed your sacral chakra for 5 to 10 breaths.
- Do the same on the other side.

Chair

- Stand up.
- Place your legs and feet together.
- As you breathe in, bend your knees as if you were going to sit.
- Raise your arms up.
- Look upwards.
- Open your root chakra for 5 to 10 breaths.

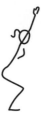

Tree

- Stand up.
- Put your palms together in front of your chest and put your weight on your right foot.
- As you breathe out, lift your perineum and tense your abs.
- Place your left foot against your right leg.
- Open your root chakra for 5 to 10 breaths and then repeat on the other side.

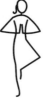

Aeroplane

- Put your bodyweight on your right foot and straighten your arms.
- As you breathe out, lift your perineum and tense your abs.
- Lean over frontwards by lifting your left leg until your body and left leg are both parallel with the floor.
- Take 5 to 10 breaths as you keep balanced.
- Do the same on the other side.

Head tap

- Sit cross-legged.
- Make your hands into fists and tap all over your scalp with your knuckles for 30 seconds.
- Concentrate on the vibrations that the tapping makes inside your head.

Moon mudra

- Sit cross-legged.
- Join the tips of your ring fingers and your thumbs.
- Put your left hand level with your stomach, with the palm facing upwards.
- Put your right hand level with your heart, palm facing down. Imagine you are stretching a thread, held between your fingers. The silver thread looks like moonlight. Welcome the feelings in your stomach and chest.

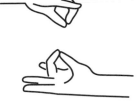

Visualisation

- Relax your hands on your knees or hips.
- Think of the moon and ask it to support your plans. Imagine a ray of moonlight that shines on you like a ray of support and agreement. Feed off this light.

Savasana

- Lie on your back for the final relaxation, with your legs stretched out in front of you and your arms beside your body with your palms facing upwards.
- Rest for 5 to 10 minutes.

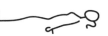

The crescent moon helps you to realise your plans. Your hair and nails grow quicker. Use facemasks and treatments in order to absorb more vitamins. Watch your figure though, as it is easy to put on weight at this time too!

Massage your solar plexus and the insides of your wrists with 1 drop of basil essential oil mixed with 5 drops of vegetable oil. The mixture will help you achieve your goals.

Wear some jewellery with lapis-lazuli in it, or carry some in your pocket to aid your creative expression.

Full moon

The full moon – like the new moon – is a phase that only lasts an instant but its effects are felt before and after it takes place (arousal, anxiety, insomnia). The full moon is a lover that reveals – and shows off – our deepest character. Like a magnifying glass, it amplifies our emotions (heart chakra), our sensitivity (sacral chakra) and our intuition (third eye chakra).

Very gentle practice is recommended in order to restore balance in the body and spirit.

Listen carefully to your body and your heart during this session; it is very likely that you will discover a new you inside.

🪷 *Note down how the full moon affects you.*

....

....

....

....

Sankalpa

· Sit down with your legs crossed.
· Put your palms together and your fingers upright together in front of your chest. Close your eyes.
· Take some deep breaths and speak your intention in a loud voice: 'I find myself and I evolve thanks to the light of the full moon.'

Torso rotation

· Place your hands on your thighs or knees.
· Rotate your body from the pelvis up. Begin with anti-clockwise rotations and then rotate clockwise.
· Open your root chakra for 5 to 10 breaths in each direction.

Inner perception

- Lie on your back with your legs straight and relaxed.
- Place your hands on your ovaries: thumbs and index fingers touching to form a triangle.
- Breathe in deeply and inflate your stomach fully and as you breathe out, deflate it.
- Open your sacral chakra for 10 to 15 breaths.

Salamander

- Lie on your front with your hands under your face.
- Relax your hips, legs and feet.
- Open your sacral chakra for 5 to 10 breaths.

Curled leaf

- Sit up.
- Spread your knees.
- Sit back on your heels and keep the tips of your toes together.
- Lower your forehead to the floor, stretch out your back and arms.
- Open your heart chakra for 5 to 10 breaths.

Crescent moon

- Get on all fours.
- Place your right foot inside your right hand.
- Anchor to the floor by bending your right knee, making sure it does not go past your ankle.
- As you breathe out, lift your perineum.
- As you breathe in, stretch your arms upwards with your palms together.
- Keep your shoulders down.
- Look straight in front of you and open your sacral chakra for 5 to 10 breaths.
- Do the same on the other side.

Sleeping swan

- Place your hands and your left knee flat on the floor in front of you, with your right leg out behind. Your left heel points to your right hand and your left knee towards your left hand.
- Lean gently forwards and put your forehead on the floor. If you cannot do that, place a cushion under your forehead. Relax your arms either side in front of you.
- Feed your heart chakra for 5 to 10 breaths.
- Repeat on the other side.

Butterfly

- Sit down.
- Bend your knees and push them towards the floor, keeping the soles of your feet together. If you feel tension in the knees, place cushions under your thighs to support your legs.
- As you breathe out, bend forwards while keeping your hands on your feet.
- Feed your sacral chakra for 5 or 10 breaths.
- Straighten your back gently.

Neck stretch

- Sit cross-legged.
- Place your hands on the opposite shoulders. Your elbows should be facing forwards and touching.
- Lower your head and look down.
- As you breathe in, push the back of your head upwards.
- Take 5 to 10 deep breaths.

Alternate breathing

- Put your left hand on your knee. Touch the space between your eyebrows with the tips of your index and middle fingers of your right hand.
- Seal your right nostril with the thumb and breathe in through your left nostril.
- Seal your left nostril with your little finger, open your right nostril and breathe out through it.

- Then breathe in through the right nostril, seal it with your thumb, release the left nostril and breathe out through the left nostril.
- Alternate your breathing for 2 to 5 cycles.

Visualisation

- Relax your hands onto your knees or hips.
- Breathe deeply, puffing yourself up each time you breathe in and relaxing as you breathe out.
- As you breathe in, earth energy flows into your body, entering via your root chakra, passing through your heart and leaving from the head.
- As you breathe out, celestial energy flows into you through the head, passing the heart and into the earth through your root chakra. Continue for 1 minute. Welcome the feelings of balance and peace that take hold.

Savasana

- Lie on your back for the final relaxation, with your legs stretched out in front of you and your arms beside your body with your palms facing upwards.
- Rest for 5 to 10 minutes.

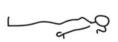

During the full moon, try not to make big decisions, as you risk being impulsive. It's time to take stock. Stay calm and take note in your diary of what is preventing you from realising your plans. Keep yourself open to revelations that will be obvious during this phase.

Take a hot bath with 10 drops of frankincense essential oil to boost self-harmony.

Carry some howlite in your pocket or hold some in your hands during meditation in order to sooth your spirit and clarify your emotions.

Waning moon

The waning moon is a period that comprises three phases and lasts 14 days. It is a period of letting go. After two weeks of growth, the waters recede and energy lowers, leading to rest.

To check it, hold your finger to the moon in a straight line down the middle. Only the left side is visible, and it forms a letter 'd' (downward).

Gentle postures encourage relaxation and are advised for the waning moon. Proceed gently and rid yourself of everything you no longer need.

🪷 *Make a note of what you would like to get rid of over the two weeks.*

....

....

....

....

....

Sankalpa

· Sit down with your legs crossed.
· Put your palms together and your fingers upright together in front of your chest. Close your eyes.
· Take some deep breaths and speak your intention in a loud voice: 'The moon is with me as I abandon all that is no longer useful to me.'

Triangle

- Stand up straight.
- Take a big step back with your right foot and turn it out to make a right angle with your left foot.
- Straighten your arms to shoulder height, keeping them parallel to the floor.
- As you breathe out, lift your perineum and keep your hips forward.
- Bend over to the left.
- Put your left hand on your shin.
- Stretch your right hand to the ceiling.
- Open your root chakra for 5 to 10 breaths.
- Do the same on the other side.

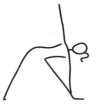

Crescent moon

- Get on all fours.
- Place your right foot inside your right hand. Anchor to the floor by bending your right knee, making sure it does not go past your ankle.
- As you breathe out, lift your perineum.
- As you breathe in, stretch your arms to the ceiling with your palms together.
- Keep your shoulders down.
- Look straight in front of you and feed your sacral chakra for 5 to 10 breaths.
- Do the same on the other side.

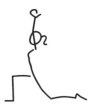

Seed

- Lie on your back.
- Bring your legs to your chest and wrap your arms around them.
- If you are not on your period, take 5 to 10 dynamic breaths: inflate your stomach as you inhale and relax it as you exhale, to the rhythm of a clock.
- Otherwise, breathe deeply and open your sacral chakra.

Supine twist

- Spread your arms out beside you as a cross.
- Bend your knees towards your chest.
- As you breathe out, move your knees to the left as you turn your head to the right. If you feel tension in your lower back, try placing a cushion under your left leg.
- Breathe deeply for 1 minute as you concentrate on your right side. Relax.
- Do the same on the other side.

Caterpillar

- Sit down with your legs out straight in front of you.
- As you breathe out, bring your upper body forwards to your legs. Keep your legs and arms relaxed.
- Open your root chakra for 5 to 10 breaths.

Feet up the wall

- Lie on your back so you can raise your legs upwards.
- Use your heels and elbows to get your bottom right up to the wall.
- Relax your arms along the sides of your body or put them on your stomach.
- Open your root chakra for 10 to 15 breaths.

Foetus

- Bend your knees and roll over to your right side.
- Put your arms under your head.
- Feed your heart chakra for 5 to 10 breaths.

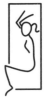

Forehead massage

- Sit cross-legged.
- Gently massage your forehead by sliding, from one side to the other, the tips of the fingers of one hand, then the other. Imagine you are chasing away the worries that were there.

Moon relaxation

- Close your eyes.
- Relax your left hand and put your right hand near your face.
- Seal your right nostril with your right thumb and close your eyes.
- Breathe deeply 5 to 10 times through your left nostril as you visualise a bright light entering and filling your energy bowl that is situated inside your hips.

Visualisation

- Lie down on your back for a body scan.
- Think about your feet and let inner peace into them. Move on to your knees, relax your calves, ankles and shins. Continue to your thighs, hips, stomach, chest, back, arms, shoulders and end at your head. Welcome the feeling of profound relaxation.

Savasana

- Lie on your back for the final relaxation, with your legs stretched out in front of you and your arms beside your body with your palms facing upwards.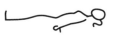
- Rest for 5 to 10 minutes.

The waning moon is the ideal time to have a big clearout. Have a detox to flush out toxins more effectively, get your hair cut – you can even make the most of this time by scheduling some depilation!

Massage the inside of your wrists with a mixture of 1 drop of melissa essential oil in 10 drops of vegetable oil to aid relaxation.

Wear a malachite jewel or carry some in your pocket, to help get rid of spent energy.

Winter

In winter, yin energy dominates nature as well as the human body.

Calm and slow are the keywords of the season. Cold weather and grey skies encourage us to keep warm and reflect upon ourselves. Winter is the ideal time to sort, to process and to let go.

A session of postures promoting internalisation and relaxation is ideal to rejuvenate you. It helps you to recharge your kidneys, which play the role of 'batteries' in traditional Chinese medicine. They are located at the level of your two lowest ribs and are linked to your root and sacral chakras.

🪷 *Note down your favourite winter relaxation activities.*

....

....

....

....

Sankalpa

· Sit down with your legs crossed.
· Put your palms together and your fingers upright together in front of your chest. Close your eyes.
· Take some deep breaths and speak your intention in a loud voice: 'I take pleasure in pampering myself.'

Salamander

· Lie on your front with your hands under your face.
· Relax your hips, legs and feet.
· If you want to, place a hot water bottle or a blanket on your lower back to recharge your kidneys.
· Open your root chakra for 5 to 10 breaths.

Tiger

- Get on all fours. Keep your knees hip width apart. Your feet should be flat on the floor and your hands should be below your shoulders.
- As you breathe in, lift your left leg up and bend your back gently.
- As you breathe out, bring the knee to the front while arching your back. Repeat 4 times on each side.
- Concentrate on the sensations in your back and your legs.

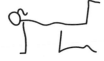
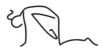

Half-butterfly

- Sit down with your left leg out in front of you.
- Bend your right knee and open it out. Your right foot should touch the inside of your left thigh.
- Curl over forwards and relax your head and arms.
- Open your root chakra for 5 to 10 breaths, then do the same on the other side.

Triskelion

- Bend your left leg so your left foot points inside.
- Bend your right leg to the outside so your right foot is behind you.
- Bend slowly over forwards, keeping your back curved and your forearms on the floor.
- Feed your kidneys for 5 to 10 breaths, then do the same on the other side.

Knee lift

- Lie on your back.
- Bring your right knee up to your chest and grasp it with your hands.
- If you are not on your period, take 5 to 10 dynamic breaths: inflate your stomach as you inhale and relax it as you exhale, to the rhythm of a clock.
- Otherwise, breathe deeply as you open your solar plexus chakra. Change to the other side.

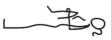

Reclining butterfly with support

· Sit down and place a bolster or rolled-up blanket at the
  base of your spine.
· Lie slowly back onto the bolster. If you feel tension in
  the neck, put a cushion under your head.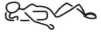
· Bend your knees and open them outwards, keeping the soles of
  your feet together.
· Place your arms alongside your body and feed your kidneys
  for 5 to 10 breaths.

Turning half-butterfly

· Put your right leg out in front of you.
· Bend your left knee and open it out. Your left foot should
  touch the inside of your right thigh.
· Put your right hand on your left thigh and lean in the direction
  of your right foot.
· Place your left arm over your head and relax it, with your elbow
  naturally bent.
· Feed your kidneys for 5 to 10 breaths.
· Do the same on the other side.

Kidney massage

· Sit cross-legged.
· Rub your hands together until you feel heat.
· Rub your lower back at kidney level for 1 minute.
· Keep your hands over your kidneys and feel the heat.

Dorsal breathing

· Stay sitting cross-legged.
· Place your hands on your knees and close your eyes.
· Breathe out, hold the breath and curl your stomach in. Keep your
  stomach in and breathe deeply for 1 minute.
· Concentrate on the feelings in the lower part of your lungs (you'll feel it
  in your back).

Visualisation

- Place your hands on your knees and imagine a ball of blue light in front of your face.
- Breathe gently and deeply as you imagine this coloured energy entering through your nostrils. It goes down into your kidneys and fills them completely. As you breathe out, let the energy settle. Do a few more breaths as you watch your kidneys fill up.

Savasana

- Lie on your back for the final relaxation, with your legs stretched out in front of you and your arms beside your body with your palms facing upwards.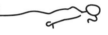
- Rest for 5 to 10 minutes.

Nature encourages us to rest during winter. The cycle of plants and animals follows it; do the same thing. Take time to rest and to pamper yourself: read on the sofa under a blanket, drink a cup of hot chocolate, have an open fire or a warm, bubbly bath. Make the most of it!

In case of ear, nose and throat sensitivities, massage your thorax and neck with a mixture of 3 drops of marjoram essential oil in 5 drops of vegetable oil.

Wear some jewellery containing fire agate, or carry some of the stone in your pocket to augment your vital strength.

Spring

In spring, nature renews the cycle of life. Happiness and hope fill our hearts. Our energy encourages new plans and new perspectives. It's a great time to detox. According to traditional Chinese medicine, spring is linked to the liver, which needs a good clean out after hibernation and the festive season.

The liver is situated at the level of your solar plexus chakra, in the upper right of the abdomen. It likes stimulation from the twisting that improves blood circulation.

🪷 *Identify the aspects of your life that are in need of a detox (body, mental, emotional, home, work etc.)*

....

....

....

....

....

Sankalpa

· Sit down with your legs crossed.
· Put your palms together and your fingers upright together in front of your chest. Close your eyes.
· Take some deep breaths and speak your intention in a loud voice: 'I rid myself of old plans and I open up to new things.'

Torso rotation

· Sit cross-legged, place your hands on your thighs or knees.
· Rotate your body from the pelvis up. Begin with anti-clockwise rotations and then rotate clockwise.
· Open your root chakra for 5 to 10 breaths in each direction.

Stretch twist

- Get on all fours.
- Put your right foot inside your right hand.
- Turn out the toes on your left foot to aid stability.
- Put your left hand on the floor inside your left foot and raise your right hand upwards.
- Stretch both hands as you push on the floor. If you are comfortable, tense your left leg.
- Look in front of you, upwards.
- Feed your solar plexus chakra for 5 to 10 breaths on each side.

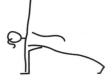

Four-limbed staff

- Stay on all fours.
- Engage your abdominal wall and turn your toes under so that they are flat on the floor.
- As you breathe out, lift your perineum. Keep your knees on the floor and bend your arms to make a right angle.
- Stretch your back. Your neck should remain straight at the top of your spine.
- Keep your shoulders down.
- If you are comfortable, lift your knees.
- Take 5 to 10 breaths and take notice of the sensations in the top of your body.

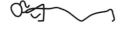

Seated twist

- Sit down with your legs out in front of you.
- Bend your right knee and place your right foot outside your left knee.
- Place your right hand on the floor behind you and your left hand on your right hip.
- As you breathe in, push yourself upwards.
- As you breathe out, turn your right shoulder behind you.
- Look over your right shoulder.
- Feed your liver for 5 to 10 breaths.
- Change to the other side and feed your solar plexus chakra.

Supine twist

- Lie down on your back.
- Put your arms out beside you as a cross.
- Bend your knees towards your chest.
- As you breathe out, move your knees to the left as you turn your head to the right. If you feel tension in your lower back, try placing a cushion under your left leg.
- Feed your liver for 5 to 10 breaths.
- Do the same on the other side and feed your solar plexus chakra.

Bridge

- Bend your knees and keep your feet hip width apart.
- Keep your arms straight by your body with your palms facing downwards.
- Breathe out, lift your perineum and push your pelvis upwards. Stay like this for 3 to 4 seconds and relax as you breathe in.
- Repeat 5 times.

False inhalation

- Put your feet on the floor and bend your knees.
- Widen your feet but keep your knees touching.
- Put your hands above your stomach.
- Breathe deeply and at the end of your outward breath hold it. Still holding your breath, open up your ribcage as if you were breathing in. Feel your stomach move. Hold for 4 to 6 seconds then breathe in.
- Repeat twice.

Eye gymnastics

- Sit cross-legged. Keep your head up straight.
- As you breathe in, look up slowly.
- As you breathe out, look down slowly.
- Repeat 3 times.
- Then as you breathe in, look to the left and as you breathe out, to the right.
- Repeat 3 times.

Liberating sound

· Put your hands on your knees or hips.
· Breathe in through your nose and, as you breathe out, pronounce 'aah' loudly.
· Repeat 2 times.

Visualisation

· Put your hands on your knees.
· Imagine a ball of green light in front of your face. Breathe gently and deeply so this coloured energy can enter through your nostrils, go down into your liver and fill it completely. As you breathe out, let the energy settle. Do a few more breaths as you watch your liver fill up with green light.

Savasana

· Lie on your back for the final relaxation, with your legs stretched out in front of you and your arms beside your body with your palms facing upwards.

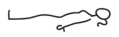

· Rest for 5 to 10 minutes.

Spring is the perfect season for a detox, including an emotional detox. Anger – the main emotion of spring according to Chinese traditional medicine – is ready to be transformed into compassion. Try the sessions on pages 126 and 208 to forgive those who are the cause.

Spray some citronella essential oil around you to help your body eliminate toxins.

Wear some jewellery containing albite, or place some of the stone on your solar plexus during lying-down meditation to help detoxify your body and spirit.

Summer

This season brings joy to your life. Women are active and ready to use the energy they have built up in the colder seasons.

Yang rules the body and spirit.

Make the most of it: move, eat seasonal fruit and vegetables and have fun.

The postures in this session will greatly stimulate the heart chakra to give you more joy and reinforce the heart, a summer organ according to Chinese traditional medicine. *Sitali* breathing will help you refresh.

🪷 *Think of lots of ways to look after yourself during the summer. Note them down here.*

....

....

....

Sankalpa

· Sit down with your legs crossed.
· Put your palms together and your fingers upright together in front of your chest. Close your eyes.
· Take some deep breaths and speak your intention in a loud voice: 'A light heart, an open spirit, I bathe in joy.'

Cow and cat

· Get on all fours with your knees hip width apart. Your feet should be relaxed and your hands should be below your shoulders.
· As you breathe in, bend your back down and look up.
· As you breathe out, arch your back and look between your knees.
· Repeat this movement 5 to 10 times as you open your heart chakra.

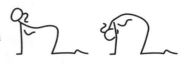

Downward-facing dog

- Hook your toes to the floor.
- As you breathe out, push the floor with your hands and toes and lift your pelvis to the ceiling. Keep your knees slightly bent in order to keep your back straight.
- Relax your head, look back between your legs.
- Open your root chakra for 5 to 10 breaths.

Cosmic dancer

- Stand up and put your bodyweight on your right foot.
- Bend your left knee.
- Put your left foot in your left hand and lift it behind you.
- Hold out your right arm horizontally, look down your right arm and bend gently forwards to keep balanced.
- Open your heart chakra for 5 to 10 breaths.
- Do the same on the other side.

Cobra

- Lie on your front.
- Keep your feet and legs together and put your hands either side of your ribcage.
- Flatten your feet and lift your perineum.
- As you breathe in, push down with your hands and lift your head, shoulders and chest. Keep your elbows bent and do not lift your shoulders.
- Look in front of you and open your heart chakra for 5 to 10 breaths.
- Put your head back down.

Bridge

- Lie on your back.
- Bend your knees with your feet hip width apart.
- Keep your arms straight by your body with your palms facing downwards.
- Breathe out, lift your perineum and push your pelvis upwards.
- Open your root chakra for 5 to 10 breaths.

Happy baby

- Bring your knees up to your chest.
- Hold the outside of your feet with your hands.
- Push your knees gently downwards, keeping your sacrum and head on the floor.
- Open your sacral chakra for 5 to 10 breaths.

Supine twist

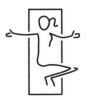

- Put your arms out beside you as a cross.
- Bend your knees towards your chest.
- As you breathe out, move your knees to the left as you turn your head to the right. If you feel tension in your lower back, try placing a cushion under your left leg.
- Breathe deeply for 1 minute as you concentrate on your right side. Relax.
- Do the same on the other side.

Thymus stimulation

- Sit cross-legged.
- Make your hands into fists.
- Tap the centre of your chest vigorously, just above your breasts, for 30 seconds.

Sitali breathing

- Put your hands on your knees or thighs.
- Stick out your tongue and roll it into a tube, pointing upwards. Keep your tongue between your lips and breathe deeply through this tube.
- Put your tongue back in and breathe gently through your nose.
- Repeat the breathing 2 times.

Visualisation

· Imagine a ball of red light in front of your face. Breath gently and deeply. The red light enters through your nostrils, goes down to your heart and fills it completely.
· As you breathe out, this energy fills your heart.
· Take some more breaths and watch your heart fill up.

Savasana

· Lie on your back for the final relaxation, with your legs stretched out in front of you and your arms beside your body with your palms facing upwards.

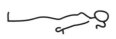

· Rest for 5 to 10 minutes.

Fire is an element that increases during the summer, causing dehydration and a lack of energy. Drink enough (water is the opposing element) and avoid sugary, fizzy drinks. Watermelon juice is perfect for cooling the body and cleansing your system.

Spray a few drops of citronella around you to keep mosquitoes away.

Wear some jewellery containing white opal, or carry some of the stone in your pocket to cool your body during a heatwave.

Autumn

This season encourages us to slow down and to reconnect with our yin energy that takes up more and more room in our body, as it does in nature. We calm down and expend less energy. The joy of summer tails off and sadness can sometimes replace it. According to Chinese traditional medicine, sadness and autumn are linked to the lungs.

The postures in this session allow the transformation of sadness into acceptance and encourage better circulation of air in the lungs to prepare for the colder season.

Think about activities that make you happy in the autumn. Note them down here.

....

....

....

....

Sankalpa

- Sit down with your legs crossed.
- Put your palms together and your fingers upright together in front of your chest. Close your eyes.
- Take some deep breaths and speak your intention in a loud voice: 'I slow down and take more time to welcome my emotions.'

Cat stretch

- Get on all fours. Keep your knees hip width apart and feet flat.
- Walk your hands forward to put your forehead on the floor.
- Open your heart chakra for 5 to 10 breaths.

Crescent moon

- Get on all fours.
- Place your right foot inside your right hand. Anchor to the floor by bending your right knee, making sure it does not go past your ankle.
- As you breathe out, lift your perineum.
- As you breathe in, stretch your arms to the ceiling with your palms together.
- Keep your shoulders down.
- Look straight in front of you and feed your heart chakra for 5 to 10 breaths.
- Do the same on the other side.

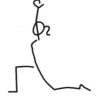

Pelvic rotation

- Stand up with your feet hip width apart.
- Put your hands on your hips.
- Make a figure of eight with your hips: 10 times one way then 10 times the other.

Dragonfly

- Sit down with your legs apart in front of you.
- Place a cushion in front of you to go beneath your upper body.
- As you breathe out, lean gently forward. Your back should be relaxed and curved.
- Open your sacral chakra for 5 to 10 breaths.

Hug

- Lie on the floor with your knees bent and together. Feet on the floor, at least hip width apart.
- Hold yourself in your arms. Stay in this position for 1 minute while breathing deeply. Whisper soft words of well-being to yourself.

Open heart

· Sit down and place a bolster or a rolled-up blanket behind your back.
· Lie down slowly on the bolster. If you feel tension in your neck, put a cushion under your head.
· Relax your arms and legs.
· Feed your lungs for 5 to 10 breaths.

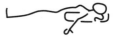

Foetus

· Bend your knees and roll over to your right side.
· Put your arms under your head.
· Feed your heart chakra for 5 to 10 breaths.

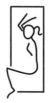

Cheek reinforcement

· Sit cross-legged.
· Breathe deeply through your nose.
· Keep some air in your mouth and puff out your cheeks.
· Move the air in your cheeks: up, left, down, right.
· Breathe out.
· Repeat 2 times and change sides.

Serpent's breath

· Put your hands by your sides.
· Breathe in through your nose and, as you breathe out, make an 'sss' sound. Your hands follow the movement of your sides.
· Repeat 2 times.

Visualisation

· Place your hands on your knees and imagine a ball of white light in front of you.
· Breathe in gently and deeply. The energy comes in through your nostrils, goes down to your lungs and fills them completely.
· As you breathe out, let this energy fill your lungs. Do a few more breaths as you watch your lungs fill up.

Savasana

· Lie on your back for the final relaxation, with your legs stretched out in front of you and your arms beside your body with your palms facing upwards.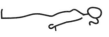
· Rest for 5 to 10 minutes.

Autumn is the season to slow down and prepare for winter. Revisit your sleep routine. Go to bed and get up one hour earlier to stay in tune with nature's changes. It will allow you to keep the energy stored in summer for longer.

Inhale a few drops of savory essential oil from a bottle or dab some between your knuckles to reinforce your immune system or to protect against viruses.

Wear some jewellery with Baltic amber in it, or carry some of the crystal in your pocket to reinforce your immune system.

—

Self-connection

An average day for a woman is often a race. This daily rush makes them forget the essential: connecting to themselves.

Devote time to yourself because self-connection gives a sense of well-being and completeness. It allows you to overcome the ups-and-downs of daily life. Connection to your body (feelings), your heart (emotions) and to your inner self (subconscious) are all necessary.

In this series you are encouraged to rest. Take a few minutes to listen to your body, your heart and your subconscious. Pay attention to what you hear.

Compassion

Compassion is innate in women. Nevertheless, women tend to spend more time looking after their nearest and dearest and their colleagues than themselves. They usually consider caring for themselves as egotistical.

According to Monique Richter, 'To be compassionate to someone means to treat them as a likeable and respectable being.'[1]

Treat yourself well; you deserve to take good care of yourself because you will later share your well-being with others. These postures of opening up your heart will help you to love and respect yourself.

🪷 *Note down how you will be good to yourself.*

....

....

....

....

Sankalpa

· Sit down with your legs crossed.
· Put your palms together and your fingers upright together in front of your chest. Close your eyes.
· Take some deep breaths and speak your intention in a loud voice: 'I love myself and I respect myself as I am.'

Foetus

· Bend your knees and roll over to your right side.
· Put your arms under your head.
· Feed your heart chakra for 5 to 10 breaths.

---

1 Monique Richter, *Petit Livre de l'auto-coaching* [*Little Book of Self-coaching*], First, 2015

Cat stretch

- Get on all fours with your knees hip width apart and your feet facing down.
- Walk your hands forward to put your forehead on the floor.
- Open your heart chakra for 5 to 10 breaths.

Tiger

- Put your hands below your shoulders.
- As you breathe in, lift your left leg up and bend your back gently.
- As you breathe out, bring the knee to the front while arching your back. Repeat 4 times on each side as you feed your heart chakra.

Locust

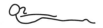

- Lie on your chest, keep your legs together and keep your front on the floor.
- Link your fingers behind your back.
- Bring your shoulder blades together, keeping your arms straight.
- As you breathe out, lift your perineum.
- Lift your head and chest, keeping your instep on the floor and pushing your hands in the direction of your feet.
- Feed your heart chakra for 5 to 10 breaths.

Inner perception

- Lie on your back with your legs straight and relaxed.
- Place your hands on your ovaries: thumbs and index fingers touching to form a triangle.
- Breathe in deeply and inflate your stomach fully.
- As you breathe out, deflate it.
- Open your sacral chakra for 10 to 15 breaths.

Hug

- Bend your knees and keep them together. Put your feet on the floor, hip width apart.
- Hold yourself in your arms.
- Feed your heart chakra for 5 to 10 breaths.

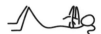

Open heart

- Sit down and place a bolster or a rolled-up blanket behind your back.
- Lie down slowly on the bolster. If you feel tension in your neck, put a cushion under your head.
- Relax your arms and legs.
- Open your heart chakra for 5 to 10 breaths.

Magic lotion

- Sit cross-legged.
- Rub the palms of your hands together until you feel heat.
- Say in a loud voice: 'I accept myself as I am. I love myself as I am. I am beautiful.'
- Place your hands on your face and imagine you are applying a cream made from love and compassion.
- Feed your face and then your hair, neck, shoulders, arms, hands and all the rest of your body to the tips of your toes.

Ganesh mudra

- Bend your elbows so your hands are at chest level.
- Put your hands so they face each other, with your left hand closer to your heart.
- Bend the fingers of your right hand and your left hand so they link together.
- Close your eyes and breathe.
- As you breathe out, pull your arms as if you wanted to separate them but do not let go.

- As you breathe in, stop pulling.
- Repeat 3 times, then change hand position: this time the right hand is closer to your heart, and repeat 3 times.
- Relax your hands onto your hips or knees and feel the sensations from your heart chakra.

Visualisation

- Imagine you are standing in front of someone you love. Concentrate on the sensations in your chest. For 30 seconds, send love and kindness to that person. Welcome the feelings. Then, imagine that person is yourself. Send yourself the same amount of love and kindness. Welcome the feelings.

Savasana

- Lie on your back for the final relaxation, with your legs stretched out in front of you and your arms beside your body with your palms facing upwards.
- Rest for 5 to 10 minutes.

Before you start your usual morning routine, look at yourself in the mirror and say some pleasant words to yourself. This may seem difficult at first, but you will soon get used to this warm welcome.

Massage your solar plexus and the inside of your wrists with a mixture of 1 drop of damask rose essential oil in 10 drops of vegetable oil. This mixture will help you to love yourself better.

Wear a chrysoprase pendant to help you stop criticising yourself.

Self-esteem and self-confidence

Self-esteem and self-confidence are linked and influence each other. Self-esteem is at the heart of our well-being. It builds from when we are children and reflects our own sense of self-value. Self-confidence is based on self-esteem becoming an action: public speaking, making new friends, making important decisions, supporting yourself etc.

This session will help you to love yourself, to awaken the courage of your solar plexus chakra and to help your self-confidence through your root chakra.

🪷 *Think of some situations where you wanted to have more self-confidence. Note them down here.*

....

....

....

Sankalpa

· Sit down with your legs crossed.
· Put your palms together and your fingers upright together in front of your chest. Close your eyes.
· Take some deep breaths and speak your intention in a loud voice: 'I have love and respect for myself and others.'

Cow and cat

· Get on all fours.
· Keep your knees hip width apart. Your feet should be flat on the floor and your hands should be below your shoulders.

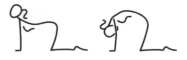

- As you breathe in, bend your back down and look up.
- As you breathe out, arch your back and look between your knees.
- Repeat this movement 5 to 10 times as you open your heart chakra.

Boat

- Sit down.
- Bend your knees and hold the backs of your thighs with your hands.
- Tense your perineum and your abdominal wall.

- As you breathe out, raise your feet one by one to have your shins parallel with the floor. If this is easy, release your hands and hold your arms out so they are parallel to the floor.
- Open your solar plexus chakra for 5 to 10 breaths.

Seated twist

- Put your left leg out in front. Bend your right knee and place your right foot outside your left knee.
- Place your right hand on the floor behind you and your left hand on your right hip.

- As you breathe in, push yourself upwards and, as you breathe out, turn your right shoulder behind you.
- Look over your right shoulder.
- If you are not on your period, take 5 to 10 dynamic breaths: inflate your stomach as you inhale and relax it as you exhale, to the rhythm of a clock.
- Otherwise, breathe deeply and open your solar plexus chakra, then change sides.

Downward-facing dog

- Get on all fours, and hook your toes to the floor.
- As you breathe out, push the floor with your hands and toes and lift your pelvis to the ceiling. Keep your knees slightly bent in order to keep your back straight.

- Relax your head, look back between your legs.
- Open your root chakra for 5 to 10 breaths.

Warrior 2

- Stand up.
- Take a big step back with your left foot and turn out your right foot to make a right angle with your left foot.
- Lift your arms so they are parallel with the floor.
- Bend your right knee but make sure it doesn't go past your ankle.
- Engage your right leg and look along the length of your left arm.
- Open your root chakra for 5 to 10 breaths.
- Do the same on the other side.

Cosmic dancer

- Stand up and put your bodyweight on your right foot.
- Bend your left knee.
- Put your left foot in your left hand and lift it behind you.
- Hold out your right arm horizontally, look down your right arm and bend gently forwards to keep balanced.
- Open your heart chakra for 5 to 10 breaths.
- Do the same on the other side.

Monkey

- Sit cross-legged with your hands on your knees.
- Put your lower lip over your upper lip.
- Lift your head, being careful with your neck. Look up or close your eyes.
- Hold for 10 seconds as you breathe deeply, then relax.
- Repeat twice.

Poise mudra

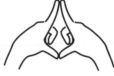

- Bend your middle fingers, ring fingers and little fingers.
- Stretch your index fingers and thumbs out as much as you can and touch the tips together.
- Close your eyes and hold the mudra in front of your solar plexus. Your thumbs should point towards the body.
- Breathe deeply for 1 minute and feel the confidence building inside you.

Visualisation

- Relax your hands on your hips or knees.
- Imagine you are starting your day and leaving the house. Each person you come across smiles nicely at you and looks admiringly at you. Welcome the sensations.

Savasana

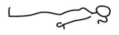

- Lie on your back for the final relaxation, with your legs stretched out in front of you and your arms beside your body with your palms facing upwards.
- Rest for 5 to 10 minutes.

Self-esteem is the image that we give back to ourselves. In order to strengthen the love that you have for yourself, make a list of your positive qualities. When you run out, ask those close to you to help you.

 Before an important event, inhale or put a few drops of cypress essential oil between your knuckles to gain more self-confidence.

Wear some jewellery containing lemon chrysoprase, or carry the crystal in your pocket or in your hands during meditation, in order to strengthen your self-esteem.

Anchoring

Our anchor is our base, our fulcrum. For humans, our anchor is the equivalent of roots for a tree and the foundations of a house. A well-anchored person feels good about themselves, has good common sense, knows their goals and gets on with their projects.

The root chakra and the small chakras in the feet help us to anchor ourselves to the earth, to feed from its powerful energy. Try this session when you feel like you need grounding, or before an important event.

🪷 *Make a note of your physical and emotional feelings after the session.*

....

....

....

....

Sankalpa

· Sit down with your legs crossed.
· Put your palms together and your fingers upright together in front of your chest. Close your eyes.
· Take some deep breaths and speak your intention in a loud voice: 'I am a woman of the earth and I am nourished by its love.'

Chair

· Stand up with your legs and feet together.
· As you breathe in, bend your knees as if you were going to sit. Raise your arms at the same time.
· Look upwards.
· Open your root chakra for 5 to 10 breaths.

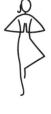

Tree

· Put your palms together in front of your chest and put your weight on your right foot.
· As you breathe out, lift your perineum and tense your abdominal wall.
· Place your left foot against your right calf.
· Open your root chakra for 5 to 10 breaths then do the same on the other side.

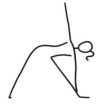

Triangle

· Take a big step back with your right foot and turn it out to make a right angle with your left foot.
· Straighten your arms at shoulder height, keeping them parallel to the floor.
· As you breathe out, lift your perineum and keep your hips forward.
· Bend over to the left and put your left hand on your shin.
· Stretch your right hand to the ceiling.
· Open your root chakra for 5 to 10 breaths.
· Do the same on the other side.

Downward-facing dog

· Get on all fours, and hook your toes to the floor.
· As you breathe out, push the floor with your hands and toes and lift your pelvis to the ceiling. Keep your knees slightly bent in order to keep your back straight.
· Relax your head, look back between your legs.
· Open your root chakra for 5 to 10 breaths.

Torso rotation

· Sit cross-legged, place your hands on your thighs or knees.
· Rotate your body from the pelvis up. Begin with anti-clockwise rotations and then rotate clockwise.
· Open your root chakra for 5 to 10 breaths in each direction.

Triskelion

· Keep your left knee bent, so your left foot points inside.
· Bend your right leg to the outside so your right foot is behind you.
· Bend slowly over your left knee and bring your forehead to the floor.
· Open your root chakra for 5 to 10 breaths.
· Do the same on the other side.

Salamander

· Lie on your front with your hands under your face.
· Relax your hips, legs and feet.
· Open your root chakra for 5 to 10 breaths.

Mouth of a fish

· Sit down cross-legged with your hands relaxed.
· Curl your lips in slightly.
· Open and close your mouth quickly, pressing your lips together like a fish.
· Repeat 9 times.

Earth mudra

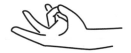

- Put your hands on your knees and touch together the tips of your thumbs and your ring fingers. The other fingers should be straight.
- Close your eyes and breathe deeply for 1 minute.
- Imagine a thread that goes from your coccyx to the centre of the earth. Welcome the sensations.

Visualisation

- Stand up with your feet hip width apart.
- Bend your knees slightly to keep your balance. Close your eyes. Concentrate on the soles of your feet. Imagine roots going from there to the centre of the earth. Breathe deeply for 1 minute, letting your used energy flow down through these roots.
- As you breathe in, inhale the nourishing energy from the earth. Keep your eyes closed for a while.

Savasana

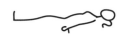

- Lie on your back for the final relaxation, with your legs stretched out in front of you and your arms beside your body with your palms facing upwards.
- Rest for 5 to 10 minutes.

Walk barefoot in grass, sand or forest as often as you can in order to activate the chakras in your feet. Also strengthen your connection with the earth by gardening.

Spray patchouli essential oil around you in order to reconnect yourself with the present moment.

Wear some jewellery containing black tourmaline, or carry the crystal in your pocket to keep your feet on the ground.

Stress relief

Overwork, family affairs and endless 'to do' lists make us weaker and more stressed. The nervous system buckles under the pressure of constant strain. This causes a weakness in the endocrine system and of the whole body. The postures in this session will help you relieve stress (throat chakra), boost your emotional stability (root chakra) and strengthen your confidence for the future (third eye chakra).

On a scale of 0 to 10 (0 being the lightest and 10 the most intense), rate your stress level. Do this again after a yoga session, and note any differences here.

....

....

....

....

....

Sankalpa

· Sit down with your legs crossed.
· Put your palms together and your fingers upright together in front of your chest. Close your eyes.
· Take some deep breaths and speak your intention in a loud voice: 'Each time I breathe out I am more relaxed.'

Aeroplane

- Stand upright with the weight of your body on your right foot and straighten your arms.
- As you breathe out, lift your perineum and tense your abdominal wall.
- Lean over forwards by lifting your left leg until your body and left leg are both parallel with the floor.
- Take 5 to 10 breaths as you keep balanced.
- Do the same on the other side.

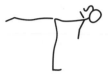

Ragdoll

- Place your feet hip width apart and bend your knees.
- As you breathe out, roll over forwards and put your chest in front of your thighs.
- Bend your elbows and hold them in your hands.
- Completely relax your upper body.
- Feed your third eye chakra for 5 to 10 breaths.

Dolphin

- Get on all fours.
- Put your forearms on the floor, keeping your elbows below your shoulders and your palms flat on the floor.
- As you breathe out, push the floor with your hands and your forearms.
- Straighten your legs as much as you feel comfortable.
- Feed your third eye chakra for 5 to 10 breaths.

Dragonfly

- Sit down with your legs apart in front of you.
- Place a cushion in front of you to go beneath your upper body.
- As you breathe out, lean gently forward. Your back should be relaxed and curved.
- Open your root chakra for 5 to 10 breaths.

Lion

- Sit on your heels.
- Widen the space between your knees, keeping your toes together, and place your palms on the floor between your knees.
- Breathe in through your nose.
- Breathe out powerfully through your mouth and stick your tongue well out. At the same time open your eyes and look at the space between your eyebrows.
- Repeat 2 times.

Bridge

- Lie on your back, and bend your knees with your feet hip width apart.
- Keep your arms straight by your body with your palms facing downwards.

- Breathe out, lift your perineum and push your pelvis upwards.
- Open your throat chakra for 5 to 10 breaths.

Feet up the wall

- Lie on your back so you can raise your legs upwards.
- Use your heels and elbows to get your bottom right up to the wall.

- Relax your arms along the sides of your body or put your hands on your stomach.
- Open your root chakra for 5 to 10 breaths.

Masseter muscles

- Sit down cross-legged.
- Place your index fingers and your middle fingers on your masseters (the muscles that move the lower jaw).
- Keep your mouth half open and massage the masseters by doing 10 circles towards the front and 10 to the back.

Time mudra

- Make fists with your hands, keeping your thumbs up.
- Put your fingers together, joining the middle knuckles with your palms facing towards you.
- Place the ends of your thumbs together
- Close your eyes and hold the mudra in front of your solar plexus as you breathe deeply for 1 minute. Become calmer little by little.

Visualisation

- Relax your hands onto your hips or knees.
- Imagine a vacuum cleaner in front of you. Let it pass all over your body to suck up all the stress and negative thoughts. Visualise this negative energy leaving your body. Welcome the feeling of lightness that enters you.

Savasana

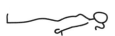

- Lie on your back for the final relaxation, with your legs stretched out in front of you and your arms beside your body with your palms facing upwards.
- Rest for 5 to 10 minutes.

Prevention is the best remedy. Often stress comes because you are overloaded. Look after yourself. Depending on what you need, try to do less each day. Make room for your priorities and delegate other tasks.

Have a bath with 10 drops of maniguette essential oil in order to relax you and help you have restful sleep.

Wear some aquamarine jewellery, or place an aquamarine on your stomach in order to balance your nervous system.

Head space and creativity

Creativity is very fulfilling. It brings a little joy to everyday life and can express itself in the way you tackle daily tasks, or in cooking or organising activities. You do not have to be an artist to be creative; everybody has their own way of doing things.

Reconnect with your source of creativity, your sacral chakra. Accept the ideas that you get from your third eye chakra. Let yourself go, and watch.

⁂ *Make a note of how you express your creativity in daily life.*

....

....

....

....

....

Sankalpa

- Sit down with your legs crossed.
- Put your palms together and your fingers upright together in front of your chest. Close your eyes.
- Take some deep breaths and speak your intention in a loud voice: 'I choose to create and I derive joy from it.'

Stretch twist

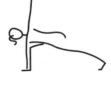

- Get on all fours and put your right foot inside your right hand.
- Turn out the toes on your left foot to aid stability.
- Put your left hand on the floor inside your left foot and raise your right hand upwards.
- Stretch both hands as you push on the floor. If you are comfortable with this, tense your left leg.
- Look in front of you, upwards.
- If you are not on your period, take 5 to 10 dynamic breaths: inflate your stomach as you inhale and relax it as you exhale, to the rhythm of a clock.
- Change to the other knee.

Downward-facing dog

- Get on all fours.
- Hook your toes to the floor.
- As you breathe out, push the floor with your hands and toes.
- Lift your pelvis to the ceiling. Keep your knees slightly bent in order to keep your back straight.
- Relax your head, look back between your legs.
- Open your third eye chakra for 5 to 10 breaths.

Garland

- Crouch down with your feet flat on the floor. If you cannot do this, place a folded blanket beneath your heels.
- Push your knees out and lean your body gently forward.
- Place your palms together in front of your chest and stretch out your back by pushing your elbows against your knees.
- If you are not on your period, take 5 to 10 dynamic breaths: inflate your stomach as you inhale and relax it as you exhale, to the rhythm of a clock.
- Otherwise, breathe deeply and feed your sacral chakra.

Swan

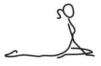

- Sit down. Bend your left knee and place your left foot in front of your right hip.
- Stretch your right leg out behind you, keeping your instep flat on the floor.
- Place your hands each side of your hips and open your chest. If you tilt to the left, place a cushion under your left buttock.
- Feed your sacral chakra for 5 to 10 breaths.
- Do the same on the other side.

Half-candle

- Lie on your back.
- Bend your knees, place your feet on the floor and your arms beside your body.
- Lift your hips and bring your knees up to your chest.
- Bend your elbows and place your hands on each side of your spine to support your lower back.
- As you breathe out, raise your legs to make an angle of roughly 60° between your legs and upper body. Your bodyweight should rest on your shoulders and arms.
- Feed your third eye chakra for 5 to 10 breaths.
- As you breathe out, bend your knees and bring your thighs towards your stomach.
- Slide your hands towards your buttocks while you gently move your back, bottom and feet to the ground.

Curled leaf

- Sit on your heels, spread your knees out and keep the tips of your toes together.
- Lower your forehead to the floor, stretch out your back and arms.
- Open your sacral chakra for 5 to 10 breaths.

Rain on the eyes

- Sit down cross-legged.
- Close your eyes for 1 minute and tap very gently on your upper and lower eyelids with the tips of your index and middle fingers.

Yoni mudra

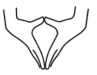

- Put together your index finger, middle finger, ring finger and little finger of each hand. Keep them straight and place them both together. Touch the tips of your thumbs and keep them far from the other fingers.
- Close your eyes and hold the mudra at lower stomach level. Your thumbs should be pointing to the sky and the other fingers to the ground.
- Breathe deeply for 1 minute. Image the mudra is a welcoming uterus that is feeding you with creative ideas.

Visualisation

- Relax your hands and put them on your hips or knees.
- Imagine you are in a pretty garden. Walk around, admire the trees, listen to the birds, smell the lovely flowers. Sit down on a bench and let your 'wise self' appear before you. It is there to help you. Ask it a question that has been bothering you and listen to the answers it gives you. Thank them for their support.

Savasana

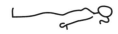

- Lie on your back for the final relaxation, with your legs stretched out in front of you and your arms beside your body with your palms facing upwards.
- Rest for 5 to 10 minutes.

To unleash your creativity, write down each morning what is going through your head, freely and without thinking. These notes are for you and by you. You will quickly notice positive changes.

Massage your lower stomach with a mixture of 5 drops of jasmine essential oil in 1 teaspoon of vegetable oil in order to boost your creativity.

Wear some jewellery containing chrysocolla, carry some in your pocket or place some on your lower stomach in order to stimulate your imagination.

Intuition

Intuition is a great quality. It is useful every day, whether choosing your path, solving problems, healing from emotional injuries more quickly or finding meaning in all that you do.

Intuition resides in the third eye chakra. This sequence of postures, and root chakra postures more generally, will help boost your intuition and keep your feet on the ground.

Listen out for what your intuition is telling you.

🪷 *Think about some situations where your intuition has helped you. Note them down here.*

....

....

....

....

Sankalpa

· Sit down with your legs crossed.
· Put your palms together and your fingers upright together in front of your chest. Close your eyes.
· Take some deep breaths and speak your intention in a loud voice: 'I am aligned with infinity.'

Warrior 2

· Stand up with your hands on your hips.
· Take a big step back with your left foot and turn it out to make a right angle with the right foot.
· Lift your arms so they are parallel with the floor.
· Bend your right knee but do not let it go past your ankle.

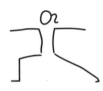

- Tense your right leg and look down under your right hand.
- Open your solar plexus chakra for 5 to 10 breaths and do the same on the other side.

Downward-facing dog

- Get on all fours, and hook your toes to the floor.
- As you breathe out, push the floor with your hands and toes and lift your pelvis to the ceiling. Keep your knees slightly bent in order to keep your back straight.
- Relax your head, look back between your legs.
- Open your solar plexus chakra for 5 to 10 breaths.

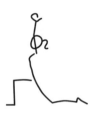

Crescent moon

- Get on all fours and place your right foot inside your right hand. Anchor to the floor by bending your right knee, making sure it does not go past your ankle.
- As you breathe out, lift your perineum.
- As you breathe in, stretch your arms to the ceiling with your palms together.
- Keep your shoulders down.
- Look straight in front of you and feed your root chakra for 5 to 10 breaths.
- Do the same on the other side.

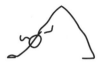

Ragdoll

- Walk your feet towards your hands.
- Place your feet hip width apart and bend your knees.
- Completely relax your upper body.
- Bend your elbows and hold them in your hands.
- Feed your third eye chakra for 5 to 10 breaths.

Sleeping swan

- Sit down.
- Bend your left knee and stretch your right leg behind you. Your left heel should be under your right hip and your left knee should face your left hand.

- Place your hands on the floor in front of you.
- Lean gently forwards and put your front on the floor. If you cannot do that, place a cushion under your front. Relax your arms either side of you.
- Feed your third eye chakra for 5 to 10 breaths.
- Repeat on the other side.

Curled leaf

- Sit on your knees and spread them out.
- Sit back on your heels and keep the tips of your toes together.

- Lower your forehead to the floor, stretch out your back and arms.
- Open your third eye chakra for 5 to 10 breaths.

Feet up the wall

- Lie on your back so you can raise your legs upwards.
- Use your heels and elbows to get your bottom right up to the wall.

- Relax your arms along the sides of your body.
- Open your third eye chakra for 5 to 10 breaths.

Third eye massage

- Sit cross-legged.
- Close your eyes and massage the point between your eyebrows with your index finger and middle finger. Start with 3 to 6 anti-clockwise circles, then do 3 to 6 clockwise circles.

Kalesvara mudra

· Put the tips of your middle fingers together.
· Bend your index fingers, ring fingers and little fingers.
  Let the knuckles touch.
· Join the tips of your thumbs together facing downwards.
  The six bent fingers and thumbs form a heart shape.
· Place the mudra in front of your forehead. Close your eyes.
· Concentrate on the space between your eyebrows.
  Breathe deeply for 1 minute.

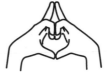

Visualisation

· Relax your hands and put them on your hips.
· Concentrate on the space between your eyebrows and imagine a beautiful
  indigo lotus there. Feed it by breathing deeply for 1 minute. Imagine the
  colour becoming more vivid and brilliant with each breath.

Savasana

· Lie on your back for the final relaxation, with your legs
  stretched out in front of you and your arms beside your
  body with your palms facing upwards.
· Rest for 5 to 10 minutes.

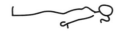

Dreams are messages sent by our subconscious.
Before you go to bed, ask your subconscious a question.
Each morning, write down your dreams in a book. Do this
as soon as you can after you wake up as we all tend to
forget our dreams very quickly.

Before meditations, put 1 or 2 drops of sandalwood essential oil on the
space between your eyebrows in order to strengthen the link with your
subconscious.

Wear a lapis-lazuli pendant or earrings, or place some under your pillow to
help enhance your intuition.

—

Emotional well-being

At the heart of well-being and balance are emotions that ebb and flow like waves. According to traditional Chinese medicine, emotions are directly linked to our bodies and any excess or shortage can directly affect our health. In order to avoid being destabilised by your emotions, choose the wave you would prefer to surf for longer without rejecting the others completely.

Grab your imaginary surf board and have fun on the waves of your emotions!

Sparking joy

Joy is a perfectly natural state of the heart, in opposition to our mental state which causes an excess of – often negative – thoughts. Joy contributes to our growth and makes us more creative, inspiring and happy. The smile is the physical manifestation of this emotion and is capable of healing the most wounded of hearts and of soothing the most painful of emotions. Arm yourself with your biggest smile.

Practise these postures to enter the world of your heart.

🪷 *Make a note of what brings you joy.*

....

....

....

....

....

Sankalpa

· Sit down with your legs crossed.
· Put your palms together and your fingers upright together in front of your chest. Close your eyes.
· Take some deep breaths and speak your intention in a loud voice: 'My heart is filled with joy and light and I will share both with others.'

Goddess

· Sit cross-legged and stretch out your arms as you breathe in.
· Look up in order to open up to joy.
· As you breathe out, put your hands on your chest to welcome the joy into your heart.
· Repeat 5 or 6 times.

Inner perception

- Lie on your back
- Put your legs out straight and relaxed.
- Place your hands on your ovaries: thumbs and index fingers touching to form a triangle.
- Breathe deeply: inflate your stomach fully as you breathe in and deflate it as you breathe out.
- Open your sacral chakra for 10 to 15 breaths.

Crescent moon

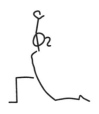

- Get on all fours.
- Place your right foot inside of your right hand. Anchor to the floor by bending your right knee, making sure it does not go past your ankle.
- As you breathe out, lift your perineum.
- As you breathe in, stretch your arms to the ceiling with your palms touching.
- Keep your shoulders down.
- Look straight in front of you and feed your heart chakra for 5 to 10 breaths.
- Do the same on the other side.

Cosmic dancer

- Stand up and put your bodyweight on your right foot.
- Bend your right knee.
- Put your left foot in your left hand and lift it behind you.
- Hold out your right arm horizontally, look down your right arm and bend gently forwards to keep balanced.
- Open your heart chakra for 5 to 10 breaths.
- Do the same on the other side.

Turning half-butterfly

- Sit down and put your right leg out in front of you.
- Bend your left knee and open it out. Your left foot should touch the inside of your right thigh.
- Put your right hand on your left thigh and lean in the direction of your right foot.
- Place your left arm over your head and relax it.
- Feed your heart chakra for 5 to 10 breaths.
- Do the same on the other side.

Happy baby

- Lie on your back and bring your knees up to your chest.
- Hold the tips of your toes with your hands.
- Push your knees downwards, keeping your sacrum and head on the floor.
- Open your sacral chakra for 5 to 10 breaths.

Open heart

- Sit down and place a bolster or a rolled-up blanket behind your back.
- Lie down slowly on the bolster. If you feel tension in your neck, put a cushion under your head.

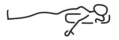

- Relax your arms and legs.
- Open your heart chakra for 5 to 10 breaths.

Binoculars

- Sit cross-legged.
- Put your hands around your eyes as if you were using binoculars.
- Apply pressure with your index fingers towards your head, just above your eyebrows. Your thumbs should rest on your cheekbones.
- Breathe deeply.
- As you breathe out, try to raise your eyebrows but press your index fingers harder to create resistance.
- Repeat 2 times.

Laughing breath

· Sit cross-legged.
· Breathe in through your nose.
· As you breathe out, do a fake laugh.
· Repeat until you actually laugh.

Visualisation

· Relax your hands onto your hips or knees.
· Close your eyes and smile.
· Breathe deeply as you smile to yourself as a sign of love and joy, for 1 minute.

Savasana

· Lie on your back for the final relaxation, with your legs stretched out in front of you and your arms beside your body with your palms facing upwards.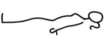
· Rest for 5 to 10 minutes.

If you really get the blues, look at yourself in a mirror and smile at yourself. Keep smiling until you feel a wave of happiness. Then continue to smile without looking in the mirror.

Spray sweet orange essential oil in order to stimulate your joy.

In order to make yourself more joyful, wear a thulite pendant or hold some in your hands as you meditate.

Depression, sadness and the blues

Sadness is an emotion that we try to escape. It can stem from our most basic needs: wanting to be loved, listened to, understood and valued. Sadness can arrive as a reaction following a happy experience (remembering great parties, summer holidays, pregnancy).

Consider the source of your grief and think about the changes you need to make to your life. Using some dynamic postures of the heart chakra you can stimulate your lungs which, according to traditional Chinese medicine, are directly linked to this emotion.

🪷 *Write down the main reason for your sadness and how you are going to alleviate it.*

....

....

....

....

....

Sankalpa

· Sit down with your legs crossed.
· Put your palms together and your fingers upright together in front of your chest. Close your eyes.
· Take some deep breaths and speak your intention in a loud voice: 'I welcome my sadness as part of my feelings.'

Warrior 1

- Take a big step backwards with your left leg and turn it outwards.
- Slowly, try to put your left heel on the floor.
- Turn your left hip to the front to keep your hips balanced.
- Bend your right knee but don't let it go further than your ankle.
- Breathe in and stretch your arms up.
- Keep your shoulders down.
- Keep looking straight in front of you and open your heart chakra for 5 to 10 breaths.
- Do the same on the other side.

Aeroplane

- Bring your feet together.
- Put the weight of your body on your right foot and straighten your arms.
- As you breathe out, lift your perineum and tense your abs.
- Lean over frontwards by lifting your left leg until your body and left leg are both parallel with the floor.
- Take 5 to 10 breaths as you maintain balance.
- Do the same on the other side.

Four-limbed staff

- Get on all fours.
- Tense your abs and tuck your toes under, onto the floor.
- As you breathe out, lift your perineum but keep your knees on the floor.
- Bend your arms to make a right angle.
- Stretch your back. Your neck should remain straight at the top of your spine.
- Keep your shoulders down. Keep your perineum engaged. If you are comfortable, lift your knees.
- Take 5 to 10 breaths and take notice of the sensations in the top half of your body.

Cobra

- Lie on your front.
- Keep your feet and legs together and put your hands either side of your ribcage. Flatten your feet and lift your perineum.
- As you breathe in, push down with your hands and lift your head, shoulders and chest. Keep your elbows slightly bent and do not lift your shoulders.
- Look in front of you and open your heart chakra for 5 to 10 breaths.
- Put your head back down.

Camel

- Sit back upright, keeping your knees and toes on the floor.
- Place your hands at the base of your back, pointing your fingers upwards.
- As you breathe in, stretch your back.
- As you breathe out, lift your perineum and tilt your pelvis forward, keeping your head upright.
- If you can, place one hand on one heel then the other on the other heel and tilt your head gently backwards. Keep your perineum engaged and your abs tensed.
- Open your heart chakra for 5 or 10 breaths.

Hug

- Lie on the floor with your knees bent but together. Feet on the floor, at least hip width apart.
- Hold yourself in your arms. Stay in this position for 1 minute while breathing deeply. Whisper soft, caring words to yourself.

Hoover

- Sit cross-legged.
- Open your mouth slightly and put your lips inside your mouth. Hold for 10 seconds as you breathe deeply through your mouth.
- Relax and repeat the breathing twice more.

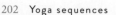

Mudra for reconnecting to your heart

- Put your left hand in the middle of your chest and the right hand on top.
- Close your eyes and breathe deeply for 1 minute. Reconnect with your heart and listen to the messages of sadness without judgement.

Visualisation

- Relax your hands on your hips or knees.
- Imagine a rucksack is stuck to your chest. It is full of sand and is so heavy that you cannot stand up straight. Take note of this feeling. Then cut a hole in the bag with imaginary scissors. The sand will flow slowly out of the bag, making you feel gradually lighter. Take the time to completely empty the bag, until you can breathe easily.

Savasana

- Lie on your back for the final relaxation, with your legs stretched out in front of you and your arms beside your body with your palms facing upwards.

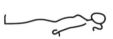

- Rest for 5 to 10 minutes.

The antidote to sadness is gratitude. It encourages optimism and gets you over the sad patches. Make a gratitude journal. Before you go to bed, write down the nice things that happened to you during the day.

 Spray some lime essential oil around you to help find emotional comfort.

Wear a serpentine crystal pendant, carry a crystal in your pocket or place it in your hands during meditation to relieve your pain.

Anxiety and fear

Fear can be useful in situations of real danger (a leap onto the pavement to avoid being hit by a car, for example). That is what we call rational fear.

There is also irrational fear, which does not bear any relation to danger and is the cause of anxiety.

According to traditional Chinese medicine, fear resides in the kidneys and manifests itself in discomfort in the stomach and chest.

Postures for the root chakra, solar plexus chakra and heart chakra can dissipate this emotion and help you find emotional security.

On a scale of 0 to 10 (0 being the least and 10 the most), evaluate and write down your anxieties. Do this again when you have finished the yoga session.

....

....

....

....

....

Sankalpa

- Sit down with your legs crossed.
- Put your palms together and your fingers upright together in front of your chest. Close your eyes.
- Take some deep breaths and speak your intention in a loud voice: 'I choose to liberate myself from the past and head to a peaceful future.

Warrior 2

- Stand up.
- Take a big step back with your left foot and turn it out to make a right angle with the right foot.
- Lift your arms so they are parallel with the floor.
- Bend your right knee but do not let it go past your ankle.
- Engage your right leg and look down the length of your right arm.
- Open your root chakra for 5 to 10 breaths.
- Do the same on the other side.

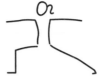

Cosmic dancer

- Stay standing up and put your bodyweight on your right foot.
- Bend your left knee.
- Put your left foot in your left hand and lift it behind you.
- Hold out your right arm horizontally, look down your right arm and bend gently forwards to keep balanced.
- Open your heart chakra for 5 to 10 breaths.
- Do the same on the other side.

Half side-plank

- Lie on your left side with your right hand on your hip.
- Place your left forearm at a right angle to the body and lean on it.
- As you breathe out, tense your abs and lift your perineum.
- Lift your hips from the floor and put your right foot on your left foot.
- If you are comfortable, lift your right hand to the ceiling.
- Open your solar plexus chakra for 5 to 10 breaths.
- Do the same on the other side.

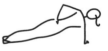

Downward-facing dog

- Get on all fours, and hook your toes to the floor.
- As you breathe out, push the floor with your hands and toes and lift your pelvis to the ceiling. Keep your knees slightly bent in order to keep your back straight.
- Relax your head, look back between your legs.
- Open your root chakra for 5 to 10 breaths.

Supine twist

- Lie down on your back.
- Put your arms out beside you as a cross.
- Bend your knees towards your chest.
- As you breathe out, move your knees to the left as you turn your head to the right. If you feel tension in your lower back, try placing a cushion under your left leg.
- Feed your solar plexus chakra for 5 to 10 breaths.
- Do the same on the other side.

Reclining butterfly with support

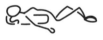

- Sit down and place a bolster or rolled-up blanket at the base of your spine.
- Lie slowly back along the bolster. If you feel tension in the neck, put a cushion under your head.
- Bend your knees and open them outwards, keeping the soles of your feet together.
- Lie your arms by your sides and channel energy to your heart chakra for 5 to 10 breaths.

Tarzan

- Sit cross-legged.
- Breathe deeply.
- Make fists with your hands. Pat the centre of your chest vigorously, just above your breasts as you make an 'aah' sound for 30 seconds.
- Repeat 2 times.

Security mudra

· Make a hollow bowl with your two hands: the left hand forms a bowl facing up, the right hand a bowl facing down.

· Close your eyes. Breathe deeply for 1 minute and imagine yourself inside the bowl. Let yourself feel the sense of security.

Visualisation

· Relax your hands on your hips or knees.

· Think of your fears or anxieties. Think of them at the level of your solar plexus. Then, breathe deeply and let the emotions escape your body like soap bubbles. Relax.

Savasana

· Lie on your back for the final relaxation, with your legs stretched out in front of you and your arms beside your body with your palms facing upwards.

· Rest for 5 to 10 minutes.

Use your inner safe place to reassure yourself. It is the place you feel safest and totally secure. It can be a real or imaginary place from your past. Take yourself there every time you feel anxiety.

Massage your solar plexus with a mixture of 2 drops of petitgrain essential oil and 4 drops of vegetable oil, to help soothe your anxieties.

Wear some jewellery with amazonite in it, carry some of the crystal in your pocket or put some on your stomach while you meditate lying down, to assuage your fears.

Anger

Anger is a strong reaction to an unwanted event or an attack on our values. Repressed anger can create tension in the body. According to Chinese traditional medicine, anger can form the basis of liver disease.

The postures in this session will help you to placate your liver (solar plexus chakra) and favour compassion and gentleness (heart chakra and sacral chakra).

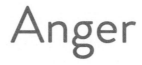 *Think of situations that make you angry. How can you prevent yourself getting angry? Note them down here.*

....

....

....

....

....

Sankalpa

· Sit down with your legs crossed.
· Put your palms together and your fingers upright together in front of your chest. Close your eyes.
· Take some deep breaths and speak your intention in a loud voice: 'I am capable of channelling my anger into something productive.'

Liberating breath

· Place your hands on your lower abdomen and form a triangle with your index fingers and thumbs.
· Inhale deeply through your nose and make yourself bigger.
· Breathe out of your mouth while making an 'aah' sound. Imagine you are breathing out your anger.

Seed

- Lie down. Bring your legs to your chest and wrap your arms around them.
- If you are not on your period, take 5 to 10 dynamic breaths: inflate your stomach as you inhale and relax it as you exhale, to the rhythm of a clock.
- Otherwise, breathe deeply and open your sacral chakra.

Turning half-butterfly

- Sit down and put your right leg out in front of you.
- Bend your left knee and open it out. Your left foot should touch the inside of your right thigh.

- Put your right hand on your left thigh and lean in the direction of your right foot.
- Place your left arm over your head and relax it, with your elbow naturally bent.
- Take 5 to 10 deep breaths. As you breathe out, do it through your mouth and make an 'aah' sound. Imagine you are breathing out all your anger.
- Do the same on the other side.

Tree

- Stand up.
- Put your palms together in front of your chest and put your weight on your right foot.

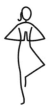

- As you breathe out, lift your perineum and tense your abs. Place your left foot against your right calf or thigh.
- Take 5 to 10 deep breaths. As you breathe out, do it through your mouth and make an 'aah' sound.
- Do the same on the other side.

Seated twist

- Sit down with your legs out in front of you.
- Bend your right knee and place your right foot outside your left knee.
- Place your right hand on the floor behind you and your left hand on your right hip.
- As you breathe in, push yourself upwards.

- As you breathe out, turn your right shoulder behind you.
- Look over your right shoulder.
- Take 5 to 10 deep breaths. As you breathe out, do it through your mouth and make an 'aah' sound.
- Repeat on the other side.

False inhalation

- Lie on your back and bend your knees. Widen your feet but keep your knees touching.
- Put your hands above your stomach.
- Breathe deeply.
- At the end of your outward breath hold it. Still holding your breath, open up your ribcage as if you were breathing in. Feel your stomach move. Hold for 4 to 6 seconds then breathe in.
- Repeat twice.

Dragonfly

- Sit down with your legs apart in front of you.
- Place a cushion in front of you to go beneath your upper body.
- As you breathe out, lean gently forward. Your back should be relaxed and curved.
- Take 5 to 10 deep breaths. As you breathe out, do it through your mouth and make an 'aah' sound.

Eyeball massage

- Sit down cross-legged and close your eyes. Put your index fingers and your middle fingers on your eyes. Without applying pressure, circle around 5 or 6 times inwards and then 5 or 6 times outwards.

Inner freedom mudra

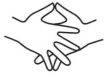

- Spread and hold out your fingers.
- Put your right hand over your left hand. Both palms should face your body.
- Slide your hands together until the index fingers and ring fingers of each hand are touching.
- Place the mudra in front of your solar plexus.
- Close your eyes and breathe deeply for 1 minute. Welcome the feeling.

Visualisation

- Relax your hands on your hips or knees.
- Think of a recent situation when you were angry. Think about what made you angry. What happened? Imagine the anger in your throat as a thick smoke. Breathe in deeply.
- As you breathe out, open your mouth and breathe hard to get all the smoke out. Repeat as many times as you need to. Welcome the feeling.

Savasana

- Lie on your back for the final relaxation, with your legs stretched out in front of you and your arms beside your body with your palms facing upwards.
- Rest for 5 to 10 minutes.

If you often have anger attacks, reconcile yourself with your past. Anger often reflects an occurrence of childhood suffering. Do not hesitate to see a specialist to help ease your suffering.

Inhale some chamomile roman essential oil from a bottle or dab a few drops between your knuckles to help anger dissipate.

Carry a rhodochrosite in your pocket, or hold some in your hands as you meditate, in order to ease conflict.

Emotional balance

An emotional imbalance often results in a rejection of unwanted emotions. The first step towards balance is to recognise your emotional state, whether it is positive or negative.

Take time to reconnect with and welcome your emotions.

Cry if you need to; it will make you feel better.

☒ *What emotions are you feeling at the moment? Write them down here.*

....

....

....

....

Sankalpa

· Sit down with your legs crossed.
· Put your palms together and your fingers upright together in front of your chest. Close your eyes.
· Take some deep breaths and speak your intention in a loud voice: 'I am in touch with all my emotions and I welcome and accept them.'

Tiger

· Get on all fours with your knees hip width apart. Your feet should be flat and your hands should be below your shoulders.
· As you breathe in, lift your left leg up and bend your back gently.
· As you breathe out, bring the knee to the front while arching your back. Repeat 4 times on each side as you feed your heart chakra.

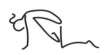

Downward-facing dog

· Hook your toes to the floor.
· As you breathe out, push the floor with your hands and toes.
· Lift your pelvis to the ceiling.
· Keep your knees slightly bent in order to keep your back straight.
· Relax your head, look back between your legs.
· Open your root chakra for 5 to 10 breaths.

Warrior 1

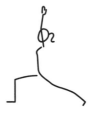

· Stand up with your hands on your hips.
· Take a big step backwards with your left leg and turn it outwards.
· Slowly, try to put your left heel on the floor.
· Turn your left hip to the front to keep your hips balanced.
· Bend your right knee but don't let it go further than your ankle.
· Breathe in and stretch your arms up, but keep your shoulders down.
· Keep looking straight in front of you and open your heart chakra.
· Do the same on the other side.

Chair

· Come to the front of the mat and straighten your legs.
· As you breathe in, bend your knees as if you were going to sit. Raise your arms at the same time.
· Look upwards.
· Open your root chakra for 5 to 10 breaths.

Triangle

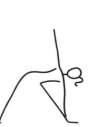

· Take a big step back with your right foot and turn it out to make a right angle with your left foot.
· Straighten your arms at shoulder height, keeping them straight and parallel to the floor.
· As you breathe out, lift your perineum.

- Bend over to the left and put your left hand on your shin, keeping your hips facing forward.
- Stretch your right hand to the ceiling.
- Open your root chakra for 5 to 10 breaths.
- Do the same on the other side.

Bridge

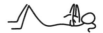

- Lie on your back, bend your knees with your feet hip width apart.
- Keep your arms straight beside your body with your palms facing downwards.
- Breathe out, lift your perineum and push your pelvis upwards.
- Feed your heart chakra for 5 to 10 breaths.

Hug

- Keep your knees bent and together. Feet on the floor, at least hip width apart.
- Hold yourself in your arms. Stay in this position for 1 minute while breathing deeply. Whisper soft words of well-being to yourself.

Eagle arms stretch

- Sit cross-legged.
- Bend your arms and place the right arm under the left.
- Place your palms together.
- Lower your head and close your eyes.
- As you breathe in, push the back of your head upwards.
- Take 5 to 10 breaths.
- Change sides, with the left arm under the right.

Alternate breathing

- Put your left hand on your knee and close your eyes.
- Touch the space between your eyebrows with the tips of your index and middle fingers of your right hand.

- Seal your right nostril with the thumb and breathe in through your left nostril.
- Seal your left nostril with your little finger, open your right nostril and breathe out through it.
- Breathe in through your right nostril, close it with your thumb, open your left nostril and breathe out through your left nostril.
- Alternate your breathing 5 times.

Visualisation

- Relax your hands on your hips or knees.
- Visualise the sea. Smell it, feel the warmth of the sun on your skin. Imagine you are surfing on waves of different sizes. They represent your emotions. You can surf every one of them. Welcome the sensation of lightness, security and happiness.

Savasana

- Lie on your back for the final relaxation, with your legs stretched out in front of you and your arms beside your body with your palms facing upwards.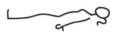
- Rest for 5 to 10 minutes.

In order to better reconnect with your emotions, ask yourself how you are feeling multiple times per day. With practice you will become more in tune with your emotions and be able to better express them.

Massage your solar plexus and spine with a mixture of 2 to 3 drops of marjoram essential oil in 10 drops of vegetable oil to calm your nerves.

Wear a lemon-turquoise gem pendant, carry some of the stone in your pocket or hold one in your hands during meditation in order to find your emotional balance.

——

Daily life

Your energy changes according to the time of day. The morning is a dynamic yang phase that peaks around midday and lowers in the afternoon. After that, passive yin takes over until bedtime. Women are influenced by these energy changes in body and spirit. Activities should be adapted to each phase.

The sessions in this section will help you stay connected to the day's natural flow and to get a good night's sleep. You can have a daily routine that benefits your body, your emotions and your femininity.

Morning

A good start sets you up well for the whole day. Morning energy is active yang energy. Make the most of this with dynamic postures that still stay connected to your female nature, yin. Efficiency, concentration and balance are your allies. You will deal with problems with ease and detachment.

Pay attention to what your body is telling you as in the morning your muscles may be tighter after a night's rest.

🪷 *What are your well-being priorities today? Write them down here.*

....

....

....

....

Sankalpa

· Sit down with your legs crossed.
· Put your palms together and your fingers upright together in front of your chest. Close your eyes.
· Take some deep breaths and speak your intention in a loud voice: 'I am ready to live a glorious day in my life.'

Goddess

· Breathe in, open your arms wide and look up.
· Breathe out, lower your head and wrap yourself in your arms.
· Repeat 5 or 6 times.

Swan

- Bend your left knee and place your left foot in front of your right hip.
- Stretch your right leg out behind you, keeping your instep flat on the floor.

- Place your hands each side of your hips and open your chest. If you tilt to the left, place a cushion under your left buttock.
- Breath deeply and visualise the air coming in and out of your chest for 5 to 10 breaths.
- Change sides.

Downward-facing dog

- Get on all fours, and hook your toes to the floor.
- As you breathe out, push the floor with your hands and toes and lift your pelvis to the ceiling. Keep your knees slightly bent in order to keep your back straight.
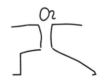
- Relax your head, look back between your legs.
- Open your solar plexus chakra for 5 to 10 breaths.

Warrior 2

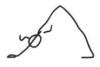
- Breathe out, put your right foot between your hands.
- Open out your left foot to make a right angle with the right foot.
- Bring your body up, bending your right knee but do not let it go past your ankle.
- Lift your arms out straight so they are parallel with the floor.
- Stretch your right leg and look along the length of your right arm.
- Take 5 to 10 breaths, lifting up your perineum each time you breathe out.
- Do the same on the other side.

Seated twist

- Sit down with your legs out in front of you.
- Bend your right knee and place your right foot outside your left knee.
- Place your right hand on the floor behind you and your left hand on your right hip.

- As you breathe in, push yourself upwards.
- As you breathe out, turn your right shoulder behind you. Look over your right shoulder.
- If you are not on your period, take 5 to 10 dynamic breaths: inflate your stomach as you inhale and relax it as you exhale, to the rhythm of a clock.
- Otherwise breathe deeply, feeding your solar plexus chakra.
  Then change sides.

Half-candle

- Lie on your back, bend your knees, place your feet on the floor and your arms beside your body.
- Lift your hips and bring your knees up to your chest. Bend your elbows and place your hands on each side of your spine to support your lower back.
- As you breathe out, raise your legs to make an angle of roughly 60°. Your bodyweight should rest on your shoulders and arms. Breathe naturally and push up and relax your perineum 21 times.
- As you breathe out, bend your knees and bring your thighs towards your stomach. Slide your hands towards your buttocks while you gently move your back, bottom and feet to the ground.

Butterfly

- Sit down, bend your knees and push them towards the floor, keeping the soles of your feet together. If you feel tension in the knees, place cushions under your thighs to support your legs.
- As you breathe out, bend forwards while keeping your hands on your feet.
- Nourish your sacral chakra for 5 or 10 breaths.
- Straighten your back gently.

Tongue to palate

- Sit cross-legged.
- Open your mouth a little a press hard on the roof of your mouth with the end of your tongue. Feel the pressure under your chin.
- Repeat the movement 5 times.

Yoni mudra

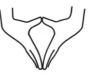

- Put together your index finger, middle finger, ring finger and little finger of each hand. Keep them straight and place them both together. Touch the tips of your thumbs and keep them far from the other fingers.
- Close your eyes and hold the mudra at lower stomach level. Your thumbs should be pointing upwards and the other fingers to the ground.
- Breathe deeply for 1 minute, welcoming the feeling in your lower stomach.

Visualisation

- Relax your hands on your knees or thighs.
- Pay attention to the space around you. Imagine a golden glow surrounding you. It protects you from unseen threats. All negative energy cannot penetrate this glow. Only positive intentions, kind words and nice people can enter. For 1 minute, concentrate on this light.

Savasana

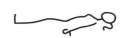

- Lie on your back for the final relaxation, with your legs stretched out in front of you and your arms beside your body with your palms facing upwards.
- Rest for 5 to 10 minutes.

The next morning starts the night before. Before you go to sleep, say to yourself: 'I will awake ready to go and in a good mood.' Day after day you will notice that getting up in the morning gets easier.

Dab a drop of verbena essential oil between your knuckles to stay calm throughout the whole day.

During the day, wear moonstone jewellery or carry a moonstone in your pocket to help you tackle your day's tasks calmly and serenely.

Afternoon

In the afternoon our energy reserves diminish.

It is usual to feel a bit tired around 4 p.m. Instead of a coffee, which only tires the body further, give yourself a bit of time to revitalise yourself with yoga.

This session is ideal for weekend afternoons as it lasts a bit longer than the others. Invite your friends to share the moment and make the most of the power of female group energy.

🪷 *Make a note of your physical and emotional sensations after the session.*

....

....

....

....

Sankalpa

· Sit down with your legs crossed.
· Put your palms together and your fingers upright together in front of your chest. Close your eyes.
· Take some deep breaths and speak your intention in a loud voice: 'I control and live my femininity. I live in my female body.'

Inner perception

· Lie on your back with your legs straight and relaxed.
· Place your hands on your ovaries: thumbs and index fingers touching to form a triangle.
· Breathe in deeply and inflate your stomach fully. As you breathe out, deflate it.
· Open your sacral chakra for 10 to 15 breaths.

Tiger

- Get on all fours with your knees hip width apart. Your feet should be flat and your hands should be below your shoulders.
- As you breathe in, lift your left leg up and bend your back gently.
- As you breathe out, bring the knee to the forehead while arching your back.
- Repeat 6 times on each side and feed your heart chakra.

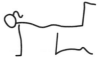
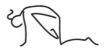

Crescent moon

- Place your right foot inside your right hand. Anchor to the floor by bending your right knee, making sure it does not go past your ankle.
- As you breathe out, lift your perineum.
- As you breathe in, stretch your arms up with your palms together.
- Keep your shoulders down.
- Look straight in front of you and feed your sacral chakra for 10 to 15 breaths.
- Do the same on the other side.

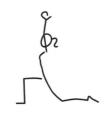

Ragdoll

- Put your hands on the floor, take a step forward on the mat.
- Place your feet hip width apart, knees bent.
- Completely relax your upper body.
- Bend your elbows and hold them in your hands.
- Take 10 to 15 deep breaths.

Supported bridge

- Lie on your back and bend your knees.
- Gently lift your hips and slide a cushion or bolster underneath.
- Widen the space between your feet and bring your knees together.
- Put your hands on your stomach.
- Breathe naturally and push up and relax your perineum 21 times.

Reclining butterfly with support

- Sit down and place a bolster or rolled-up blanket at the base of your spine.
- Lie slowly back along the bolster. If you feel tension in the neck, put a cushion under your head.
- Bend your knees and open them outwards, keeping the soles of your feet together.
- Put your hands on your stomach and nourish your ovaries and your uterus for 10 to 15 breaths.

Foetus

- Bend your knees and roll over to your right side.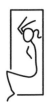
- Put your arms under your head.
- Feed your heart chakra for 10 to 15 breaths.

Full massage

- Sit cross-legged.
- Rub your palms together until you feel warmth.
- Massage the trapezius muscles (where the shoulders meet the neck) by sliding your hands from back to front for 1 minute.
- Massage your scalp with the tips of your fingers.
- Massage your forehead: slide your hands from one side to the other.
- Massage your cheeks and eyelids: place your palms on your cheeks with the tips of your fingers touching your eyebrows and slide towards your temples.
- Finish with a neck massage: slide your hands from your chin to your collarbones.

Consciousness mudra

- Put your hands on your knees or thighs.
- Touch the tips of your index fingers and thumbs.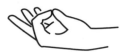
- Close your eyes and breathe deeply for 1 minute. Welcome the sensation of calm and inner peace.

Visualisation

- Relax your fingers.
- Focus on the parts of you that are touching the floor and turn your attention to your coccyx. Imagine a shining red light there. This is your root chakra. Breathe deeply for 1 minute. Each time you breathe in, the light that enters goes down to your root chakra and fills it. Move your attention to your sacral chakra, which is orange and at the level of your lower stomach. Feed it for 1 minute. Continue on to your solar plexus chakra, which is yellow, your heart chakra, which is green and at the centre of your chest, and your blue throat chakra. Finally go up to your indigo third eye chakra and your white crown chakra at the top of your head. Spend another minute imagining all your chakras shining internally and externally. Welcome the feelings.

Savasana

- Lie on your back for the final relaxation, with your legs stretched out in front of you and your arms beside your body with your palms facing upwards.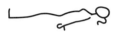
- Rest for 5 to 10 minutes.

If you have planned an activity that requires a lot of attention, try not to eat a big meal beforehand.
A stomach that is too full requires a lot of energy to digest and causes a slowdown in brain activity.

 During the session, spray rose essential oil around you to reconnect with your femininity.

If you are tired, wear a red garnet bracelet or carry a garnet in your pocket to boost your energy levels.

Evening

In order to start the day on the right foot you should make sure you sleep well. Stress creates muscular tension which stops you getting to sleep quickly and prevents deep sleep.

The postures and techniques in this session will help you to relax your muscles and to calm your busy spirit. Leave your worries outside your yoga mat and make the most of the moment.

🪷 *Think of the moments you are proud of in your day. Note them down here.*

....

....

....

....

....

Sankalpa

· Sit down with your legs crossed.
· Put your palms together and your fingers upright together in front of your chest. Close your eyes.
· Take some deep breaths and speak your intention in a loud voice: 'I am ready for today, and its highs and lows.'

Salamander

· Lie on your front with your hands under your face.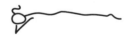
· Relax your hips, legs and feet.
· Breathe out through your mouth, making an 'aaah' sound. Imagine you are breathing out your used energy (pain, tension, tiredness, negative thoughts etc).

Garland

- Crouch down with your feet flat on the floor.
- Place a folded blanket beneath your heels if you need to.
- Push your knees out and lean your body gently forward.
- Stretch out your back by pushing your elbows against your knees.
- Feed your sacral chakra for 5 to 10 breaths.

Torso rotation

- Sit cross-legged, place your hands on your thighs.
- Rotate your body from the pelvis up. Begin with anti-clockwise rotations and then rotate clockwise.
- Open your root chakra for 5 to 10 breaths in each direction.

Dragonfly

- Place your legs apart in front of you.
- Place a cushion in front of you to go beneath your upper body.
- As you breathe out, lean gently forward. Your back should be relaxed and curved.
- Open your sacral chakra for 5 to 10 breaths.

Turning half-butterfly

- Keep your right leg out in front of you, bend your left knee and open it out. Your left foot should touch the inside of your right thigh.
- Put your right hand on your left thigh and lean in the direction of your right foot.
- Place your left arm over your head and relax it.
- Feed your heart chakra for 5 to 10 breaths.
- Do the same on the other side.

Supine twist

- Lie down on your back with your arms out beside you as a cross.
- Bend your knees towards your chest.
- As you breathe out, move your knees to the left as you turn your head to the right. If you feel tension in your lower back, try placing a cushion under your left leg.
- Breathe deeply for 1 minute as you concentrate on your right side. Relax.
- Do the same on the other side.

Feet up the wall

- Lie on your back so you can raise your legs upwards.
- Use your heels and elbows to get your bottom right up to the wall.
- Relax your arms along the sides of your body.
- Open your root chakra for 10 to 15 breaths.

Ear massage

- Sit cross-legged.
- For 1 minute, pinch each part of your ears between your index fingers and thumbs.

Moon breathing

- Close your eyes, relax your left hand and keep your right hand close to your face.
- Block your right nostril with your right thumb and close your eyes.
- Take 5 to 10 deep breaths through your left nostril.
- Visualise the clear, brilliant light that is entering your left nostril and filling your entire body.

Visualisation

· Relax your hands.

· Imagine you are sitting on a beach in front of a beautiful sunset. You can feel warm sand between your toes, the breeze on your skin and you can smell the 'iodine' odour of the sea. The sun gives the sky a red-orange hue. The more the sun goes down behind the horizon the more relaxed you feel. Once the sun has completely disappeared you are completely relaxed.

Savasana

· Lie on your back for the final relaxation, with your legs stretched out in front of you and your arms beside your body with your palms facing upwards.

· Rest for 5 to 10 minutes.

In order to get better sleep, give yourself a night-time routine. The golden rule is to switch off all electronic devices (computers, laptop, TV) at least one hour before you go to bed. The light from those screens stimulates your brain and prevents sleep.

Before you go to bed, massage your solar plexus with 2 drops of lavender essential oil to help you sleep better.

Place an amethyst under your pillow to encourage sweet dreams.

Intense day

Transport problems, work emergency, a difficult interview, dropping something, forgetting… We've all had a day when nothing goes right.

Days like these are part of life. Unfortunately, it is usually those nearest to us who bear the brunt of our anger and frustration.

If you get the chance, spend some time on your yoga mat when you get home. You can free yourself from your anger and have a much more pleasant evening.

🪷 On a scale of 0 to 10 (0 being the lowest and 10 the highest), evaluate and write down your stress level. Do the same thing after a yoga session.

....

....

....

....

....

Sankalpa

· Sit down with your legs crossed.
· Put your palms together and your fingers upright together in front of your chest. Close your eyes.
· Take some deep breaths and speak your intention in a loud voice: 'I welcome and appreciate the lessons I learned today.'

Anti-stress breathing

· Breathe deeply through the nose and purse your lips as though whistling.
· Breathe out gently, keeping your lips pursed. Take longer breathing out than breathing in.
· Continue 5 to 10 times. You stress level lowers with each outward breath.

Curled leaf

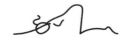

- Sit back on your heels with your knees spread out and the tips of your toes touching.
- Lower your forehead to the floor, stretch out your back and arms.
- Open your sacral chakra for 5 to 10 breaths.

Cat stretch

- Get on all fours, knees hip width apart and insteps of your feet facing the floor.
- Walk your hands forward to put your forehead on the floor.
- Open your heart chakra for 5 to 10 breaths.

Ragdoll

- Stand up.
- Place your feet hip width apart.
- Bend your knees and completely relax your upper body.
- Bend your elbows and hold them in your hands.
- Take 10 to 15 deep breaths.

Lion

- Sit on your heels, widen the space between your knees, keeping your toes together.
- Place your palms on the floor between your knees.
- Breathe in through your nose. Breathe out powerfully through your mouth and stick your tongue well out. At the same time open your eyes and look at the space between your eyebrows.
- Repeat two more times.

Triskelion

- Bend your left leg so your left foot points inside.
- Bend your right leg to the outside so your right foot is behind you.
- Bend over slowly, keeping your back rounded and your forearms on the floor.
- Open your third eye chakra for 5 to 10 breaths.
- Do the same on the other side.

Open heart

- Sit down and place a bolster or a rolled-up blanket behind your back.
- Lie down slowly on the bolster. If you feel tension in your neck, put a cushion under your head.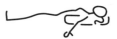
- Relax your arms and legs.
- Open your heart chakra for 5 to 10 breaths.

Palming

- Sit cross-legged.
- Rub your palms together until you feel heat.
- Cup your hands over your closed eyes.
- Lower your head and breathe deeply for 1 minute. Relax your eyelids and eyeballs.

Mudra kali

- Interlace your fingers, apart from your two index fingers which you point together. Cross your left thumb over your right.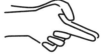
- Place the mudra over your shins or your feet, pointing the index fingers towards the floor.
- Close your eyes and imagine that your worries and tiredness from the day are leaving through your index fingers in a cloud of dark smoke. Little by little the colour becomes clearer and you feel a lightness take hold.
- Hold the mudra while breathing deeply for 1 minute.
- Thank the earth for transforming the used energy into positive energy.

Visualisation

- Keeping your eyes closed, relax your hands.
- Stay sitting down, hugging yourself in your arms.
- Lower your head. Stay in this position for 1 minute, breathing deeply and whispering gentle, comforting words to yourself.

Savasana

- Lie on your back for the final relaxation, with your legs stretched out in front of you and your arms beside your body with your palms facing upwards.
- Rest for 5 to 10 minutes.

At work, before a meeting or any stressful situation, find a quiet place and do some anti-stress breathing. This breathing stimulates your parasympathetic system which helps us handle stress by keeping us in a calm and relaxed state.

Take a warm bath with 10 drops of frankincense essential oil to get rid of the stresses of the day.

Hold some rhyolite in your hands during meditation in order to give you a positive outlook on life.

Table of benefits: dynamic yang postures

Aeroplane (root chakra and solar plexus chakra)	· Improves balance and concentration. · Strengthens calves, ankles, knees and thighs. · Stimulates the abdominals. · Opens up the ribcage. · Calms the mind.
Boat (solar plexus chakra)	· Tones abdominals, back and thighs. Helps weight loss. · Improves digestion. · Activates self-confidence and sense of power.
Bridge/dynamic bridge (throat chakra)	· Improves breathing. · Aids suppleness of spine. Strengthens thighs. · Stimulates thyroid and parathyroid glands. · Stabilises mood swings. Facilitates self-expression.
Camel (heart chakra)	· Improves respiration. · Stretches thighs and abdominals. · Aids spinal suppleness. Massages abdominal organs. Stimulates thyroid and parathyroid glands. · Aids self-expression. Heals emotional pain. Eliminates fear.
Chair (root chakra and solar plexus chakra)	· Strengthen thighs, ankles, knees and back. · Opens up the ribcage. Stimulates abdominal organs. · Encourages a sense of power.
Cobra (root chakra, sacral chakra and heart chakra)	· Improves breathing, digestion and elimination of toxins. · Strengthens the back and abdominals. Aids spinal suppleness. · Helps with good posture. Massages abdominal organs: stimulates kidneys, liver, pancreas and ovaries. · Heals emotional pain. Develops positive spirit.
Cosmic dancer (root chakra, sacral chakra, solar plexus chakra, heart chakra)	· Improves balance, breathing and concentration. · Strengthens calves, ankles, knees and thighs. · Stimulates digestive organs and sends blood to kidneys and adrenal glands. · Banishes fear.
Dolphin (root chakra and third eye chakra)	· Strengthens muscles in arms, chest, legs and back. · Opens ribcage and shoulders. Sends oxygen to brain, face and scalp. · Encourages bravery.
Downward-facing dog (root chakra and third eye chakra)	· Stimulates entire body. Tones and stretches back, arm and leg muscles. · Strengthens heart. Sends oxygen to the brain, face and scalp for anti-ageing effects. · Calms the nervous system.

Fish (throat chakra)	· Improves breathing. · Aids suppleness of spine. Stimulates thyroid and parathyroid glands. · Eliminates stress and emotional trauma. Facilitates self-expression. Heals emotional pain.
Four-limbed staff (root chakra, solar plexus chakra)	· Strengthens chest, back, buttocks, thighs and abdominals. · Develops good posture. · Boosts vital energy. Improves self-confidence.

Half-candle
(throat chakra)
	· Encourages suppleness in throat and spine.
	· Increases blood flow to skin. Sends oxygen to brain.
	  Relieves heavy legs, heals haemorrhoids and varicose veins.
	· Prevents prolapse. Stimulates thyroid and parathyroid glands, pituitary
	  gland, pineal gland.
	· Balances nervous system. Develops patience and emotional stability.
	  Facilitates self-expression.

Half side-plank (solar plexus chakra)	· Strengthens abdominals, chest, arms, back and legs. · Stimulates abdominal organs. Helps weight loss. · Increases vital energy.
Lion (throat chakra)	· Relieves tension in neck and jaw. · Activates thyroid and parathyroid glands. Improves appetite. Boosts vital energy. · Liberates unspoken and used energy accumulated in the throat. · Facilitates self-expression. Releases anger.
Locust (root chakra, sacral chakra, heart chakra)	· Reinforces back and abdominal muscles. · Develops good posture. Massages abdominal organs. Stimulates kidneys, liver and ovaries. · Improves digestion and elimination. · Heals emotional pain. Eliminates fear. Improves creativity.
Pelvic rotation (root chakra and sacral chakra)	· Aids suppleness of hips and lower back. · Improves lower back blood circulation. · Helps reconnection to feminine energy by improving blood flow to the ovaries and uterus.
Plough (throat chakra)	· Strengthen spine and kidneys. · Massages internal organs. Stimulates pancreas, thyroid and parathyroid glands, pituitary gland, pineal gland. · Boosts vital energy. Aids self-expression.
Seated twist (root chakra, sacral chakra, solar plexus chakra)	· Increases suppleness of spine and shoulders. · Massages abdominal organs, pancreas, ovaries and pelvic organs. · Facilitates detox. Stimulates the stomach and accelerates the evacuation of abdominal fat · Helps with letting go.

Stretch twist (sacral chakra and solar plexus chakra)	· Improves balance, concentration and elimination of toxins. · Strengthens legs and arms. · Opens up ribcage and shoulders. · Encourages suppleness in spine and neck. Massages abdominal organs, pancreas and ovaries. · Increases energy circulation in pelvis. Boosts vital energy.
Tiger (heart chakra)	· Improves breathing. · Strengthens back and buttocks. · Increases suppleness of spine and hips. Massages abdominal organs. · Gives a sensation of space in your heart energy.
Tree (root chakra)	· Improves balance and concentration. · Strengthens calves, ankles, knees and thighs. · Calms the spirit.
Triangle (root chakra, solar plexus chakra)	· Strengthens ankles, legs, back and arms. · Opens up ribcage and shoulders. · Gives a sense of stability and security. Encourages inner strength.
Warrior 1 (root chakra and solar plexus chakra)	· Reinforces and firms legs, arms and back. Opens up hips. Stretches shoulders, neck and arms. · Mental calmness. Increases self-confidence. Awakens the warrior spirit.
Warrior 2 (root chakra and solar plexus chakra)	· Reinforces and firms legs, arms and back. Stretches muscles in thighs, calves, shoulders and neck. · Improves breathing, concentration and oxygenation. · Develops healthy self-perception.

Relaxing yin postures

Bridge with support (sacral chakra, heart chakra)	· Loosens lower back. · Improves blood circulation around the heart. · Improves digestion. · Rebalances the nervous system. · Stimulates ovaries. Strengthens the conscious energy circulation in the pelvis. · Relieves period pain and heals illness in reproductive organs. · Soothes the mind. Removes anxieties.
Butterfly/half-butterfly (root chakra, sacral chakra)	· Opens hips. Stretches inner thighs. Loosens back. · Improves blood and energy circulation in the pelvis. · Relieves period pain and heals illness in reproductive organs. Activates feminine energy. · Facilitates letting go and emotional cleansing. Reconnection to your self. Gives a feeling of security and rootedness.
Cat stretch (heart chakra, third eye chakra)	· Improves breathing. · Encourages suppleness of spine. Improves posture. Stretches shoulders and armpits. · Reactivates feminine yin energy. · Banishes fear. Relieves stress.

Caterpillar (root chakra, sacral chakra)	· Loosens the back. Stretches back of thighs. · Improves blood and energy circulation in the lower body. Stimulates kidneys and stomach. · Massages ovaries. Reactivates feminine yin energy. · Facilitates letting go and emotional cleansing. Reconnection to the self. Gives a sensation of rootedness.
Child (sacral chakra and third eye chakra)	· Stretches back and buttock muscles. · Massages internal organs. Improves digestion. · Rebalances nervous system. · Soothes the mind. Removes anxiety. Gives a sensation of inner peace.
Cow and cat (heart chakra, throat chakra)	· Encourages suppleness of spine and neck. Improves posture. Opens rib cage. · Massages internal organs. Stimulates thyroid and parathyroid glands. · Helps letting go and reducing stress.
Crescent moon (sacral chakra, solar plexus chakra, heart chakra)	· Improves breathing. · Stretches groin and psoas muscle. Encourages suppleness of shoulders, neck and arms. Stimulates energy in the spine and *Sushumna* channel. · Reduces stress and fear. Reconnection to lunar energy.
Curled leaf (root chakra, sacral chakra, heart chakra, third eye chakra)	· Opens up hips. Loosens lower back. Stretches back, shoulders and armpits. · Relieves period pain and heals illness in reproductive organs. Activates feminine energy. · Rebalances nervous system. · Full relaxation. Soothes the spirit.
Dragonfly (root chakra, sacral chakra)	· Stretches thighs. · Improves blood and energy circulation in the pelvis. Massages ovaries. Relieves period pain and heals illness in reproductive organs. · Facilitates letting go and emotional cleansing. Reconnection to your self. Gives a feeling of rootedness.
False inhalation (solar plexus chakra)	· Stimulates digestive organs. Reduces excess of intestinal gas. Facilitates detox. · Stimulates ovaries. · Improves concentration. Calms the spirit.
Feet up the wall (root chakra)	· Improves sleep. · Rebalances the nervous system. Irrigates the brain. · Improves blood circulation around the heart. · Relieves heavy legs, heals haemorrhoids and varicose veins. · Gives a sensation of inner security. Soothes the mind.
Foetus (heart chakra)	· Rebalances the nervous system. Improves blood circulation to the entire body. · Gives a sensation of comfort. Reconnection to maternal love.
Garland (root chakra, sacral chakra)	· Opens the pelvis; encourages hip flexibility. Relaxes spine and neck. · Stimulates stomach and improves elimination. · Improves energy circulation in pelvis. Stimulates the ovaries. Relieves period pain and heals illness in reproductive organs. Activates feminine energy. Reconnection to femininity. · Soothes the spirit. Gives a feeling of security.

Goddess (heart chakra)	· Improves breathing and posture. · Encourages suppleness of spine. Stretches the neck. · Gives a sensation of fulfilment and joy. Reinforces self-esteem and self-confidence. Awakens your inner goddess.
Happy baby (sacral chakra)	· Opens up the pelvis. Decompresses the lumbar region. Stretches insides of thighs and the spine. · Improves energy circulation in the pelvis. Massages ovaries. Relieves period pain and heals illness in reproductive organs. Reactivates feminine yin energy. · Eliminates fear and anger. Reconnects you to your inner child.
Hug (heart chakra)	· Stretches arm muscles. · Reactivates feminine yin energy. · Soothes the spirit. Gives inner peace. Facilitates acceptance of weaknesses. Reinforces self-esteem.
Inner perception (sacral chakra)	· Rebalances nervous system. Improves circulation. · Strengthens the conscious energy circulation in the pelvis. Relieves period pain and heals illness in reproductive organs. Stimulates the ovaries and uterus. Activates feminine energy. · Soothes the mind. Removes anxiety. Improves creativity.
Knee lift (sacral chakra)	· Stretches the buttocks and arms. · Massages internal organs. Improves digestion and reduces excess of gas. · Reduces tiredness. · Reactivates feminine yin energy. · Facilitates letting go. Calms the nervous system. Soothes the mind.
Open heart (heart chakra)	· Improves breathing, sleep and energy circulation at heart level. · Rebalances the nervous system. · Banishes fear. Gives sensation of fulfilment. · Reactivates feminine yin energy.
Ragdoll (third eye chakra, crown chakra)	· Loosens back muscles. Stretches spine and neck. · Oxygenates the skin. Sends oxygen to the brain. · Stimulates thyroid and parathyroid glands, pituitary gland, pineal gland. · Facilitates letting go. Eliminates stress.
Reclining butterfly (sacral chakra)	· Opens hips. Stretches inner thighs. · Improves blood and energy circulation in the pelvis and legs. Stimulates ovaries. Relieves period pain and heals illness in reproductive organs. Activates feminine energy. · Reconnection to your femininity. Calms agitated mind.
Reclining butterfly with support (sacral chakra, heart chakra)	· Improves breathing and sleeping. · Opens hips. Stretches inner thighs. · Improves blood and energy circulation in the pelvis and legs. Stimulates ovaries. Relieves period pain and heals illness in reproductive organs. Activates feminine energy. · Banishes fear. Reduces stress.
Rest (root chakra, heart chakra)	· Relieves lower back. Relaxes the psoas, the muscles that connect the hips and lumbar region. · Reactivates feminine yin energy. · Calms the spirit.

Salamander (root chakra)	· Rebalances nervous system. Improves circulation. · Relieves period pain and heals illness in reproductive organs. · Calms the mind. Removes anxiety. Reinforces our bond with the earth. Gives a feeling of security and rootedness.
Savasana (all chakras)	· Deep relaxation of all muscles. Regenerating. · Reduces tiredness. Calms agitated spirit. Gives a feeling of inner peace.
Seed (sacral chakra)	· Stretches buttocks and legs. · Massages intestines, ovaries and uterus. Improves digestion and reduces excess gas. · Reactivates feminine yin energy. · Facilitates letting go. Calms the nervous system. Soothes mental agitation.
Sleeping swan (root chakra, sacral chakra, third eye chakra)	· Stretches buttocks and opens up hips. Loosens back. · Stimulates ovaries. Improves circulation in the pelvis. Relieves period pain and heals illness in reproductive organs. · Gives a feeling of security and peace.
Supine twist (sacral chakra, solar plexus chakra, heart chakra)	· Stretches the spine. Encourages suppleness of hips and shoulders. · Massages kidneys and liver. Stimulates the stomach and accelerates the evacuation of abdominal fat. · Rebalances the nervous system. · Reactivates feminine yin energy. Rebalances masculine and feminine energy.
Swan (root chakra, sacral chakra, heart chakra)	· Improves breathing. · Stretches buttocks and opens up hips. Encourages suppleness of spine. · Stimulates abdominal organs. · Reactivates feminine yin energy. · Releases stress. Gives a sensation of security and peace.
Torso rotation (root chakra, sacral chakra)	· Encourages suppleness of hips and lumbar region. · Improves circulation in the lower body. · Strengthens anchoring. · Reconnects to feminine energy. Encourages blood flow to ovaries and uterus.
Triskelion (root chakra, sacral chakra)	· Opens up hips. Encourages suppleness in spine. Massages ovaries. · Improves digestion and reduces intestinal gas. · Improves blood and energy circulation in the pelvis. Relieves period pain and heals illness in reproductive organs. Stimulates the ovaries and uterus. Activates feminine yin energy. · Reconnection to your self. Facilitates relaxation.
Turning half-butterfly (root chakra, heart chakra)	· Improves breathing. · Encourages suppleness of spine. Stretches armpits. Massages kidneys and liver. · Eliminates negative emotions. Gives a sensation of security and rootedness. Reactivates feminine yin energy.

Acknowledgements

This book is the fruit of much collaboration. I would therefore like to thank all of the brilliant people who accompanied me on this project.

Thank you to Agnès Vidalie, editor, friend, pupil, for your support and encouragement through the entire process.

Enormous gratitude to my editors: Aline Sibony for the trust she had in me, and Cyrielle Londero for her professionalism and editorial advice. Thank you to you both for being there.

Thank you to Iris Glon for creating such beautiful illustrations of the yoga poses.

A big thank you to my dear friend, yoga teacher Julie Brion, for transforming my words into comprehensible language.

To Élodie Garamond of the Tigre Yoga Club for the inspiration and trust she gives me.

To my dear friends Ricarda and Éric Langevin of the Yoga Vision studio for their support and encouragement for all these years.

I am grateful to all my teachers for the knowledge they have passed to me and to all my students – it is thanks to them that Yoga for Women has evolved.

And thank you to you, lovely women, for existing, for loving your sacred femininity and for shining your light and living your lives in the world.

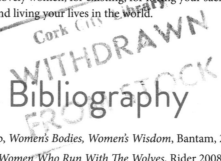

Bibliography

Dr Christiane Northrup, *Women's Bodies, Women's Wisdom*, Bantam, 2010

Clarissa Pinkola Estes, *Women Who Run With The Wolves*, Rider 2008

Cyndi Dale, *The Subtle Body*, Sounds True 2009

Dr Danièle Flaumenbaum, *Woman Desired, Woman Desiring*, Aeon Books 2020

Dr Françoise Barbira Freedman, *Yoga for Pregnancy, Birth and Beyond*, Dorling Kindersley 2020

Gertrud Hirschi, *Mudras: Yoga In Your Hands*, Coronet 2016

Maisie Hill, *Period Power*, Bloomsbury 2018

Nicola Jane Hobbs, *Thrive Through Yoga*, Bloomsbury 2017

Sally Kempton, *Awakening Shakti*, Sounds True 2013

Lama Tsultrim Allione, *Wisdom Rising*, Atria/Enliven Books 2018

Uma Dinsmore-Tuli, *Yoni Shakti*, Pinter & Martin 2014